Development of the Pancreas and Neonatal Diabetes

Endocrine Development

Vol. 12

Series Editor

P. Mullis Bern

1st ESPE Advanced Seminar in Developmental Endocrinology,
Paris, May 10–11, 2007

Development of the Pancreas and Neonatal Diabetes

Volume Editors

R. Scharfmann Paris

J.P.H. Shield Bristol

21 figures, 11 in color, and 9 tables, 2007

KARGER

Basel · Freiburg · Paris · London · New York ·
Bangalore · Bangkok · Singapore · Tokyo · Sydney

Endocrine Development
Founded 1999 by Martin O. Savage, London

Raphael Scharfmann
Hôpital Necker
INSERM U845
Paris, France

Julian P. Hamilton-Shield
University of Bristol and
Bristol Royal Hospital for Children
Bristol, UK

Library of Congress Cataloging-in-Publication Data

ESPE Advanced Seminar in Developmental Endocrinology (1st : 2007 : Paris)
Development of the pancreas and neonatal diabetes / volume editors, R. Scharfmann, J.P.H. Shield.
p. ; cm. – (Endocrine development, ISSN 1421-7082 ; v. 12)
At head of title: 1st ESPE Advanced Seminar in Developmental Endocrinology, Paris, May 10–11, 2007.
Includes bibliographical references and indexes.
ISBN-13: 978-3-8055-8385-5 (hardcover : alk. paper)
1. Diabetes in children–Congresses. 2. Newborn infants–Diseases–Congresses. 3. Pancreas–Growth–Congresses. 4. Pancreas–Pathophysiology–Congresses. I. Scharfmann, R. (Raphael) II. Shield, J.P.H. (Julian P.H.) III. Title. IV. Series.
[DNLM: 1. Pancreas–embryology–Congresses. 2. Diabetes Mellitus–diagnosis–Congresses. 3. Diabetes Mellitus–therapy–Congresses. 4. Infant, Newborn–Congresses. W1 EN3635 v.12 2007 / WI 800 E77d 2007]
RJ520.D5E77 2007
618.92'462–dc22

2007031802

Bibliographic Indices. This publication is listed in bibliographic services, including Current Contents® and PubMed/MEDLINE.

Disclaimer. The statements, options and data contained in this publication are solely those of the individual authors and contributors and not of the publisher and the editor(s). The appearance of advertisements in the book is not a warranty, endorsement, or approval of the products or services advertised or of their effectiveness, quality or safety. The publisher and the editor(s) disclaim responsibility for any injury to persons or property resulting from any ideas, methods, instructions or products referred to in the content or advertisements.

Drug Dosage. The authors and the publisher have exerted every effort to ensure that drug selection and dosage set forth in this text are in accord with current recommendations and practice at the time of publication. However, in view of ongoing research, changes in government regulations, and the constant flow of information relating to drug therapy and drug reactions, the reader is urged to check the package insert for each drug for any change in indications and dosage and for added warnings and precautions. This is particularly important when the recommended agent is a new and/or infrequently employed drug.

www.karger.com
Printed in Switzerland on acid-free and non-aging paper by Reinhardt Druck, Basel
ISSN 1421–7082
ISBN 978–3–8055–8385–5

Contents

Preface

The European Society for Paediatric Endocrinology (ESPE) is at the forefront of research and training for paediatric endocrinologists across Europe. Much of adult disease as well as conditions treated in childhood have their basis in fetal and early childhood development and growth. In May 2007 in Paris, ESPE organised and funded its first, 2-day symposium on developmental biology, bringing together scientists and clinicians to discuss and evaluate what is known on pancreatic development and its implications for human disease and treatment. Both experts and postgraduate students attended in the expectation that this would generate new research ideas for future paediatric-based studies. The meeting, generously supported by Novo Nordisk, Lilly and Ipsen, was a great success and the level of scientific discussion of high calibre.

In this volume, we have asked the speakers at the symposium to produce monographs based on their lectures. The chapters include, amongst others, work on human and animal pancreatic developmental biology, imprinting, genetics and the investigation, management and treatment of neonatal diabetes and congenital hyperinsulinaemia. This collection should prove of interest to endocrinologists, geneticists and pancreatic developmental scientists alike.

Raphael Scharfmann, Paris
Julian Hamilton-Shield, Bristol

Shield JPH, Scharfmann R (eds): Development of the Pancreas and Neonatal Diabetes.
Endocr Dev. Basel, Karger, 2007, vol 12, pp 1–11

Pancreatic Development as a Basis for the Definition of New Therapies for Diabetes

Raphael Scharfmann

INSERM U845, Necker Hospital, Faculty of Medicine, University Paris-Descartes, Paris, France

Abstract

Understanding pancreas development is important for at least 3 reasons: first, from a cognitive point of view, to understand the development of a complex organ, the pancreas; next, because it is now clear that abnormal pancreas development can give rise to specific forms of diabetes in humans, and finally, because if we want to define new treatments for diabetes based on cell therapy or regenerative medicine, we will have to understand in detail how β-cells develop. In this chapter, I will rapidly summarize what we currently know concerning pancreas development. I will next try to demonstrate that cell replacement therapy for diabetes requires a near-perfect understanding of how β-cells develop.

Type 1 and type 2 diabetes mellitus (T1DM and T2DM) are chronic diseases, which are currently suboptimally treated and cannot be cured. The diseases affect more than 10 million Europeans and their treatment is predicted soon to consume as much as 10% of the health care budgets of many westernized societies. The lack of adequate treatment modalities results, at least in part, from the absence of a detailed understanding of the molecular mechanisms underlying the development of such diseases which in turn limits our capacity to develop drugs targeting the most relevant physiological dysfunctions. Both T1DM and T2DM are characterized by insufficient insulin secretion related to the demand. In T1DM, insulin-producing cells are destroyed, while in T2DM there is a dysfunction of the insulin-secreting pancreatic β-cells and a relative decrease in insulin action on target tissues such as muscle, fat and liver. There is now strong evidence that the reduced insulin secretion capacity of the endocrine pancreas may be a primary cause of T2DM development. This reduced secretion capacity may be caused either by a progressive insensitivity of the β-cells to elevations in blood glucose concentrations and/or by a reduction in the total β-cell mass [1].

It can easily be postulated that understanding the physiology of β-cell mass development represents a necessary step to better understand the pathophysiology of diabetes and to progress in the definition of new treatments or a cure for diabetes. This point is supported by at least 3 examples: (1) the demonstration in 1994 that the pancreas did not develop in mice deficient for the transcription factor Ipf1/Pdx1 [2], leading to the identification of a cause of pancreatic agenesis in humans [3]; (2) progress in the definition of the crucial role of the ATP-sensitive potassium channel for insulin secretion by pancreatic β-cells [4] that led to the description of ABCC8, which encodes one of the proteins of the ATP-sensitive potassium channel present in β-cells, being mutated in patients with neonatal diabetes [5]; on the basis of these results, treatment with sulfonylureas was initiated in patients with permanent neonatal diabetes and transient neonatal diabetes and has proved effective [5]; (3) it now seems certain that production from embryonic stem cells (ES cells) of human β-cells to be used for therapeutic purposes will require a near-perfect understanding of the way β-cells form during normal development [6].

In this chapter, I will briefly review our current knowledge concerning pancreas development, a topic that will be described in detail by Martin et al. [this vol., pp. 24–32] in another chapter of this book. I will next present different experiments performed in various laboratories and use the conclusions of such studies as a basis to demonstrate that it is crucial to perfectly understand how β-cells develop if we are to define new therapies for diabetes based on either cell replacement therapy or through regenerative medicine.

Pancreatic Development

The mature pancreas contains two types of tissue: endocrine islets composed of cells that produce hormones such as insulin (β-cells), glucagon (α-cells) somatostatin (Δ-cells), pancreatic polypeptide (PP-cells) and ghrelin (ε-cells), and exocrine tissue composed of acinar cells that produce enzymes (e.g. carboxypeptidase A) secreted via the pancreatic ducts into the intestine [7–11]. The pancreas originates from the dorsal and ventral regions of the foregut endoderm directly posterior to the stomach. Over the last few years, important findings have shed light on the processes controlling pancreatic endocrine cell development. Studies of genetically engineered mice identified a hierarchy of transcription factors regulating pancreas organogenesis and islet cell differentiation [12–17]. The endodermal region committed to pancreatic development first expresses the homeodomain-containing transcription factor *Pdx1* (pancreatic duodenal homeobox-1). *Pdx1* is detected in mouse embryos on embryonic day 8.5 (E8.5; E9 in rats, 5 weeks of development in humans) in early pancreatic progenitor cells [18–20]. During adulthood, *Pdx1* expression becomes largely confined to the β-cells, where it activates insulin gene transcription [19]. Targeted disruption of the *Pdx1* gene in mice leads to pancreatic agenesis [21, 22]. Interestingly, in 1997, Stoffers et al. [3] reported a case of a young patient with pancreatic agenesis. It was found that this patient was homozygous for a single nucleotide deletion of the human *Pdx1* gene, whereas both parents are heterozygotes for the same mutation. The deletion was not found in normal individuals, strongly suggesting that Pdx1 is necessary for pancreas development in humans. Taken together, these data indicate that *Pdx1* is necessary for the morphogenesis and differentiation of the pancreatic buds both in rodents and humans [3]. *Pdx1* is also an efficient marker of early pancreatic progenitor cells.

Differentiation into endocrine and exocrine cells is the next step during this process of differentiation, and cell tracing experiments have shown that both endocrine and exocrine cells derive from *Pdx1*-expressing progenitor cells [23, 24]. The basic helix-loop-helix transcription factor neurogenin 3 *(Ngn3)* is expressed in epithelial pancreatic progenitor cells prior to endocrine differentiation and is subsequently downregulated during differentiation [25]. *Ngn3* is necessary for pancreatic endocrine cell development, and *Ngn3*-deficient mice lack pancreatic endocrine cells [26]. Lineage tracing experiments have provided direct evidence that *Ngn3*-expressing cells are islet progenitors [23]. Thus, *Ngn3* is a marker of choice for detecting the onset of pancreatic endocrine cell differentiation. It was reasonable to speculate that Ngn3 should play the same role in rodents and humans and thus patients with mutations giving rise to lack of function of Ngn3 should be born diabetic without endocrine cells in their pancreas. However, a recent study showed that people with mutations in Ngn3 have significant congenital, malabsorptive diarrhea, but are not diabetic at birth. Importantly, this loss-of-function mutation was described as giving rise to an inactive form of Ngn3 [27]. Based on such results, it was speculated that in humans, as is the case in rodents, Ngn3 would play a major role in the development and function of intestinal cells [27, 28]. On the other hand, it seemed that Ngn3 was necessary for β-cell development in rodents, but not in humans [26, 27]. However, this last hypothesis was not supported by recent data indicating that the described mutation [27] was not null, but hypomorphic, and capable of inducing endocrine development when expressed in the primitive gut endoderm of chicken embryo [29].

Finally, the pancreatic phenotype of patients and rodents with mutations in the POU-homeobox TCF2 (vHNF1, HNF1β) gene is also interesting. In both rodents and humans, mutations in this gene result in pancreas atrophy or agenesis [30–34]. Thus, it seems that the same set of transcription factors control pancreas development in both rodents and humans.

Whereas information is accumulating on the transcriptional control of pancreatic development, little is known about the mechanisms by which extracellular signals control the expression of the relevant genes. Pancreas differentiation is controlled by permissive signals derived from adjacent mesodermal structures. Specifically, at early stages of development, signals from the notochord in direct contact with the endodermal region that will develop into pancreas [35–37] control the first steps of pancreatic development. Later on (around E8.5 in mice), signals from the dorsal aorta are crucial for proper pancreatic development [38–41]. And finally, signals from the mesenchyme, which condenses around the underlying committed endoderm, control the subsequent steps [8]. Classic explant culture experiments highlighted the importance of the mesenchyme for exocrine pancreas growth and differentiation [42, 43]. However, the role of the mesenchyme in regulating β-cell mass remained unclear. For example, results based on loss of function of genes encoding growth factors expressed in the pancreatic mesenchyme, such as fibroblast growth factor 10 (FGF10), suggest that signals from the mesenchyme directly and positively control the final number of β-cells [44]. On the other hand, when the same growth factor was overexpressed in the pancreas, β-cell development was inhibited [45, 46]. Thus, the exact effect of mesenchymal signals on β-cell development remained controversial, as studies of loss and gain of FGF10 function suggest opposite conclusions. However, by using an in vitro culture model on rat embryonic pancreas, it was clearly shown recently that FGF10 was able to amplify pancreatic progenitor cells, giving rise to an increase in the final number of β-cells that develop [47].

In conclusion, we begin to have a clear picture of transcription factors and intercellular signals important for proper pancreatic development.

β-Cell Production from Different Tissue Sources

Over the last few years, different cell types have been tested for their potential to differentiate into β-cells. The rationale here was the following one: in 2000, an important clinical study performed by a Canadian team was published indicating that by using the right protocol (now called 'the Edmonton protocol'), patients with T1DM could be cured following a graft of human pancreatic islets derived from cadaveric donors [48]. This work was a major advance in this field but had a number of limitations that have recently been clearly described [49]. One such important limitation is the few available islet donors when compared to the high number of potential recipients. It is thus clear that alternative sources of β-cells have to be defined.

Xenotransplantation as a Source of New β-Cells

One approach is to use islets from animals and perform xenotransplantation. Interestingly, the morphological characteristics, the ability to respond to glucose challenge and the cell composition of human and pig islets are very similar. Moreover, pig differs from human insulin in only one amino acid and not so long ago, diabetic patients were treated with insulin prepared from pig pancreatic extracts. However, immune rejection remains a major problem with grafting pig islets into diabetic patients, but genetically modified pigs have been generated to reduce the immunological reactivity of humans to porcine tissue [50].

β-Cell Generation by Transdifferentiation

A second approach is to generate β-cells from tissues that normally do not produce insulin by a mechanism that would not mimic normal β-cell development but would resemble transdifferentiation. In this context, different groups have tried to generate β-cells from hematopoietic stem cells or from liver cells. The example of β-cell differentiation from hematopoietic stem cells is extremely interesting. In fact, at the end of the last century, an impressive quantity of scientific reports were published indicating that when bone marrow or fractions enriched in hematopoietic stem cells were grafted into mice, lung, gut, skin, myoblast, hepatic and neuroectodermal cells of donor origin could be found in the recipient animal [51–57]. Such results were in my opinion very surprising. The extensive published literature in prestigious, scientific journals seemed to indicate that hematopoietic stem cells had the capacity to differentiate into nearly all cell types and in 2003 a publication appeared in the *Journal of Clinical Investigation* entitled: 'In vivo derivation of glucose-competent pancreatic endocrine cells from bone marrow without evidence of cell fusion' [58]. The results of this work indicated that adult mouse bone marrow contains cells that can differentiate into pancreatic β-cells. These bone marrow-derived cells, once engrafted into the pancreatic islets of their host, exhibited markers and physiological behavior characteristic of pancreatic β-cells: they expressed and secreted insulin upon glucose stimulation. Moreover, transdifferentiation of bone marrow cells into β-cells was proposed as being a frequent event based on the fact that 4–6 weeks after bone marrow transplantation, 2–3% of the β-cells found in the islets were derived from the bone marrow. An editorial was also written entitled: 'Bone marrow: an extra-pancreatic hideout for the elusive pancreatic stem cell?' [59]. At that juncture, the question was whether other groups could reproduce such impressive and unexpected results. During the past few years, three independent groups tried to reproduce such results without success [60–62]. Thus at that point, the consensus was that hematopoietic stem cells do not differentiate into pancreatic β-cells. In fact, it is also interesting to note that the general interest of scientists around the world in transdifferentiation of hematopoietic stem cells into nonhematopoietic cells has strongly decreased and it can be proposed that a large number of results that appeared on transdifferentiation have been overinterpreted. However, there is possibly one important piece of information in such studies. An interesting study published a few years ago indicates that bone marrow-derived stem cells can initiate pancreatic regeneration [63]. In this study, the authors injected adult bone marrow-derived cells into mice whose β-cells had been destroyed with streptozotocin. However, here bone marrow-derived cells migrated to the pancreas but did not differentiate into β-cells. Instead, they became vascular endothelial cells and increased the vascularity of the pancreas. Thus, in this case, the mechanism would not be based on transdifferentiation, but on the traditional framework of germ layer specification in which bone marrow stem cells differentiate into endothelial cells [64]. Such results fit well with data presented above indicating that during embryonic life, signals from endothelial cells have a permissive effect on pancreatic cell differentiation [38–41]. However, the exact mechanism by which endothelium would induce β-cell regeneration during adult life needs now to be dissected in detail. The major questions are: do endothelial signals activate the proliferation of β-cells that escape streptozotocin destruction or do β-cells develop under such conditions in the adult pancreas following a mechanism that recapitulates the major steps of β-cell differentiation that occur in vivo? Cell tracing experiments in recently engineered mice should permit to answer this type of questions [65].

Differentiation of liver cells into β-cells has also represented a major topic of research with the goal of producing new sources of β-cells. It is known that during embryonic life, bipotential precursors exit in the gut endoderm that have the potential to differentiate into pancreatic and liver cells [66]. During the past few years, researchers have thus tried to define protocols to generate β-cells from liver cells from different species such as frog, rodent or human [67–73]. The first paper on this topic was published in 2000 and since then a number of laboratories in the world have focused on this topic which remains potentially interesting.

β-Cell Development from ES Cells

During the past few years, different groups have examined the possibility of producing β-cells from ES cells. ES cells were interesting based on their almost unlimited proliferation capabilities and their potential to differentiate into cells of the 3 primary cell layers. One of the first publications was by Soria et al. [74] who used a cell-trapping system to select mouse ES cells able to transcribe the insulin gene. Once implanted in the spleen of diabetic mice, such cells corrected hyperglycemia. This work was important because it demonstrated that mouse ES cells can develop into insulin-transcribing cells. Lumelsky et al. [75] next designed a new protocol to generate in vitro insulin-containing cells from mouse ES cells. They developed a specific protocol to differentiate β-like cells from mouse ES cells. Importantly, this protocol did not recapitulate the major steps of development that occur during β-cell differentiation, but was based on the enrichment of nestin-positive cells, which represent progenitors for neuronal cells [76]. At that time, it was thought that nestin was also a marker of pancreatic progenitor cells [77]. However, more recent work does not support this hypothesis [78–81]. Lumelsky et al. [75] were able to show that the β-like cells they developed from mouse ES cells secreted insulin by a mechanism that resembles the one found in mature pancreatic β-cells, but when grafted into diabetic mice, glycemic levels did not decrease. Next, two groups further modified the in vitro protocol. Hori et al. [82] treated mouse ES cells with inhibitors of phosphoinositide 3-kinase. They were able to generate cells that contained insulin at levels far greater than previously reported. Moreover, transplantation of such cells to diabetic mice improved glycemic control and completely rescued survival [82]. Blyszczuk et al. [83] transfected mouse ES cells with Pax4, a transcription factor known to be necessary in vivo for β-cell development [84]. They demonstrated that under such conditions, the development of insulin-producing cells was promoted and based on such work, insulin-positive cells containing granules typical of adult β-cells were produced. Transplantation of these cells into diabetic mice normalized blood glucose levels for at least 2 weeks [83]. At that point, such results indicated that insulin-containing cells that resemble pancreatic β-cells could be generated from mouse ES cells. In some studies, such cells responded to glucose in terms of insulin secretion and produced enough insulin to normalize blood glucose levels when grafted into diabetic mice. Cell tumorogenicity was also analyzed. It is indeed known that undifferentiated or partially differentiated ES cell grafts often form tumors. It was shown that when mouse ES cells were treated with inhibitors of phosphoinositide 3-kinase, no tumor was detected for 8 weeks after cell transplantation [82]. Some of the rodent data described above were tested in human ES cells and it was shown that human ES cells could differentiate and produce insulin. Taken together, the data described above indicate that using a specific protocol, a large fraction of ES cells can differentiate into insulin-producing cells that resemble β-cells.

However, some of the studies presented above have some limitations. First, when insulin content per cell was measured it was quite low when compared to insulin content per β-cell. Next, in the 2 cases where hyperglycemia was normalized by grafting insulin-producing cells derived from ES cells, the graft was not removed at the end of the experiment to definitively demonstrate that glycemic levels were controlled by the grafted cells [74, 83]. Some of this work has recently been challenged. While it was shown that insulin-positive cells could be detected by immunocytochemistry when ES cells were grown in culture, it was quite clearly demonstrated that the vast majority of the cells did not effectively produce insulin. Based on different experimental arguments, it was proposed that the vast majority of insulin-positive cells would have absorbed insulin present in the culture medium, while only extremely rare cells (1/100,000) would in fact transcribe the insulin gene [85]. While this last work was highly convincing and reproduced by another team [86], it does not explain how in 3 different studies ES cells had a beneficial effect when grafted into diabetic mice [74, 82, 83]. Thus, at that point, no reproducible protocol was available to generate β-cells from ES cells. The field is now possibly progressing rapidly with a recent work strongly suggesting that β-cells can be generated from human ES cells. In this study, the authors have designed a multistep protocol that tries to reproduce in a culture dish the major steps of β-cell development: formation of definitive endoderm, followed by gut tube formation, by posterior foregut formation, by pancreatic endoderm and endocrine precursor development and finally by hormone-expressing endocrine cells [87]. In a previous work published by the same group, the authors had described a protocol to produce definitive endoderm from human ES cells [88] and in the new study the authors added 4 additional steps. The cells produced at the end of the protocol had similarities and differences when compared to human β-cells. For example, their insulin content was not so different from the one found in normal β-cells and the cells secreted insulin upon depolarization [87]. However, a large number of insulin-expressing cells produced with this protocol also expressed glucagon, which is not the case for mature β-cells found in the pancreas. Moreover, the cells did not secrete insulin upon glucose stimulation. While the authors were optimistic and suggested they had developed not yet fully differentiated β-cells that had the potential to differentiate into mature β-cells, the arguments to support this hypothesis were weak. In conclusion, while this latest work that tried to mimic in vitro the way β-cells develop in vivo represents a major step forward in progress when compared to what had previously been done, it can be postulated that key information is still lacking to generate fully mature human β-cells.

Conclusion

During the past few years, we have learned a lot concerning the way β-cells develop during prenatal life. We have also learned that the best way to produce in vitro β-cells from ES cells is to replicate the physiological development of β-cells [6]. This therefore requires a perfect understanding of the way β-cells develop. We are beginning to have a clear picture of transcription factors and intercellular signals important for proper pancreatic development, but it is also clear that some information is missing before we are confidently able to generate β-cells from ES cells.

Acknowledgements

Work in our laboratory is supported by INSERM-JDRF Grant (AIP Cellules Souches A03139MS), the 6th European Union Framework Program (Beta-Cell Therapy Integrated Project), the Institut National de la Santé et de la Recherche Médicale/Fondation pour la Recherche Médicale/Juvenile Diabetes Research Foundation (Grant 4DA03H), the French National Program of Research on Diabetes, and the Association Française des Diabétiques.

References

1 Butler AE, Janson J, Bonner-Weir S, Ritzel R, Rizza RA, Butler PC: Beta-cell deficit and increased beta-cell apoptosis in humans with type 2 diabetes. Diabetes 2003;52:102–110.

2 Jonsson J, Carlsson L, Edlund T, Edlund H: Insulin-promoter-factor I is required for pancreas development in mice. Nature 1994;371:606–609.

3 Stoffers DA, Zinkin NT, Stanojevic V, Clarke WL, Habener JF: Pancreatic agenesis attributable to a single nucleotide deletion in the human IPF1 gene coding sequence. Nat Genet 1997;15:106–110.

4 Aguilar-Bryan L, Bryan J: Molecular biology of adenosine triphosphate-sensitive potassium channels. Endocr Rev 1999;20:101–135.

5 Babenko AP, Polak M, Cave H, Busiah K, Czernichow P, Scharfmann R, Bryan J, Aguilar-Bryan L, Vaxillaire M, Froguel P: Activating mutations in the ABCC8 gene in neonatal diabetes mellitus. N Engl J Med 2006;355:456–466.

6 Madsen OD, Serup P: Towards cell therapy for diabetes. Nat Biotechnol 2006;24:1481–1483.

7 Heller RS, Jenny M, Collombat P, Mansouri A, Tomasetto C, Madsen OD, Mellitzer G, Gradwohl G, Serup P: Genetic determinants of pancreatic epsilon-cell development. Dev Biol 2005;286:217–224.

8 Pictet R, Rutter W: Development of the embryonic pancreas; in Steines DF, Frenkel N (eds): Handbook of Physiology. Baltimore, Williams & Wilkins Co, 1972, vol 1, pp 25–66.

9 Prado CL, Pugh-Bernard AE, Elghazi L, Sosa-Pineda B, Sussel L: Ghrelin cells replace insulin-producing beta cells in two mouse models of pancreas development. Proc Natl Acad Sci USA 2004;101: 2924–2929.

10 Scharfmann R: Control of early development of the pancreas in rodents and humans: implications of signals from the mesenchyme. Diabetologia 2000; 43:1083–1092.

11 Slack J: Developmental biology of the pancreas. Development 1995;121:1569–1580.

12 Collombat P, Hecksher-Sorensen J, Serup P, Mansouri A: Specifying pancreatic endocrine cell fates. Mech Dev 2006;123:501–512.

13 Edlund H: Pancreas: how to get there from the gut? Curr Opin Cell Biol 1999;11:663–668.

14 Edlund H: Organogenesis: pancreatic organogenesis developmental mechanisms and implications for therapy. Nat Rev Genet 2002;3:524–532.

15 Murtaugh LC: Pancreas and beta-cell development: from the actual to the possible. Development 2007; 134:427–438.

16 Murtaugh LC, Melton DA: Genes, signals, and lineages in pancreas development. Annu Rev Cell Dev Biol 2003;19:71–89.

17 Wilson ME, Scheel D, German MS: Gene expression cascades in pancreatic development. Mech Dev 2003;120:65–80.

18 Jensen J, Heller RS, Funder-Nielsen T, Pedersen EE, Lindsell C, Weinmaster G, Madsen OD, Serup P: Independent development of pancreatic alpha- and beta-cells from neurogenin3-expressing precursors: a role for the notch pathway in repression of premature differentiation. Diabetes 2000;49:163–176.

19 Ohlsson H, Karlsson K, Edlund T: IPF1, a homeodomain-containing transactivator of the insulin gene. EMBO J 1993;12:4251–4259.

20 Piper K, Brickwood S, Turnpenny LW, Cameron IT, Ball SG, Wilson DI, Hanley NA: Beta cell differentiation during early human pancreas development. J Endocrinol 2004;181:11–23.

21 Ahlgren U, Jonsson J, Edlund H: The morphogenesis of the pancreatic mesenchyme is uncoupled from that of the pancreatic epithelium in IPF1/PDX1-deficient mice. Development 1996;122: 1409–1416.

22 Offield M, Jetton T, Laborsky P, Ray M, Stein R, Magnuson M, Hogan B, Wright C: PDX-1 is required for pancreatic outgrowth and differentiation of the rostral duodenum. Development 1996; 122:983–995.

23 Gu G, Dubauskaite J, Melton DA: Direct evidence for the pancreatic lineage: NGN3+ cells are islet progenitors and are distinct from duct progenitors. Development 2002;129:2447–2457.

24 Herrera PL: Adult insulin- and glucagon-producing cells differentiate from two independent cell lineages. Development 2000;127:2317–2322.

25 Apelqvist A, Li H, Sommer L, Beatus P, Anderson DJ, Honjo T, Hrabe de Angelis M, Lendahl U, Edlund H: Notch signalling controls pancreatic cell differentiation. Nature 1999;400:877–881.

26 Gradwohl G, Dierich A, LeMeur M, Guillemot F: Neurogenin3 is required for the development of the four endocrine cell lineages of the pancreas. Proc Natl Acad Sci USA 2000;97:1607–1611.

27 Wang J, Cortina G, Wu SV, Tran R, Cho JH, Tsai MJ, Bailey TJ, Jamrich M, Ament ME, Treem WR, et al: Mutant neurogenin-3 in congenital malabsorptive diarrhea. N Engl J Med 2006;355:270–280.

28 Jenny M, Uhl C, Roche C, Duluc I, Guillermin V, Guillemot F, Jensen J, Kedinger M, Gradwohl G: Neurogenin3 is differentially required for endocrine cell fate specification in the intestinal and gastric epithelium. EMBO J 2002;21:6338–6347.

29 Jensen JN, Rosenberg LC, Hecksher-Sorensen J, Serup P: Comment on: Mutant neurogenin-3 in congenital malabsorptive diarrhea. N Engl J Med 2007; 356:1781–1782.

30 Baeyens L, Bonne S, German MS, Ravassard P, Heimberg H, Bouwens L: Ngn3 expression during postnatal in vitro beta cell neogenesis induced by the JAK/STAT pathway. Cell Death Differ 2006;13: 1892–1899.

31 Barbacci E, Chalkiadaki A, Masdeu C, Haumaitre C, Lokmane L, Loirat C, Cloarec S, Talianidis I, Bellanne-Chantelot C, Cereghini S: HNF1beta/TCF2 mutations impair transactivation potential through altered co-regulator recruitment. Hum Mol Genet 2004;13:3139–3149.

32 Bellanne-Chantelot C, Chauveau D, Gautier JF, Dubois-Laforgue D, Clauin S, Beaufils S, Wilhelm JM, Boitard C, Noel LH, Velho G, Timsit J: Clinical spectrum associated with hepatocyte nuclear factor-1beta mutations. Ann Intern Med 2004;140: 510–517.

33 Haumaitre C, Barbacci E, Jenny M, Ott MO, Gradwohl G, Cereghini S: Lack of TCF2/vHNF1 in mice leads to pancreas agenesis. Proc Natl Acad Sci USA 2005;102:1490–1495.

34 Haumaitre C, Fabre M, Cormier S, Baumann C, Delezoide AL, Cereghini S: Severe pancreas hypoplasia and multicystic renal dysplasia in two human fetuses carrying novel HNF1beta/MODY5 mutations. Hum Mol Genet 2006;15:2363–2375.

35 Hebrok M, Kim SK, St Jacques B, McMahon AP, Melton DA: Regulation of pancreas development by hedgehog signaling. Development 2000;127:4905–4913.

36 Kim S, Hebrok M, Melton D: Notochord to endoderm signaling is required for pancreas development. Development 1997;124:4243–4252.

37 Kim SK, Hebrok M: Intercellular signals regulating pancreas development and function. Genes Dev 2001;15:111–127.
38 Jacquemin P, Yoshitomi H, Kashima Y, Rousseau GG, Lemaigre FP, Zaret KS: An endothelial-mesenchymal relay pathway regulates early phases of pancreas development. Dev Biol 2006;290:189–199.
39 Lammert E, Cleaver O, Melton D: Induction of pancreatic differentiation by signals from blood vessels. Science 2001;294:564–567.
40 Lammert E, Cleaver O, Melton D: Role of endothelial cells in early pancreas and liver development. Mech Dev 2003;120:59–64.
41 Yoshitomi H, Zaret KS: Endothelial cell interactions initiate dorsal pancreas development by selectively inducing the transcription factor Ptf1a. Development 2004;131:807–817.
42 Golosow N, Grobstein C: Epitheliomesenchymal interaction in pancreatic morphogenesis. Dev Biol 1962;4:242–255.
43 Wessels N, Cohen J: Early pancreas organogenesis: morphogenesis, tissue interactions, and mass effects. Dev Biol 1967;15:237–270.
44 Bhushan A, Itoh N, Kato S, Thiery J, Czernichow P, Bellusci S, Scharfmann R: Fgf10 is essential for maintaining the proliferative capacity of epithelial progenitor cells during early pancreatic organogenesis. Development 2001;128:5109–5117.
45 Hart A, Papadopoulou S, Edlund H: Fgf10 maintains notch activation, stimulates proliferation, and blocks differentiation of pancreatic epithelial cells. Dev Dyn 2003;228:185–193.
46 Norgaard GA, Jensen JN, Jensen J: FGF10 signaling maintains the pancreatic progenitor cell state revealing a novel role of Notch in organ development. Dev Biol 2003;264:323–338.
47 Attali M, Stetsyuk V, Basmaciogullari A, Aiello V, Zanta-Boussif MA, Duvillie B, Scharfmann R: Control of beta-cell differentiation by the pancreatic mesenchyme. Diabetes 2007;56:1248–1258.
48 Shapiro AM, Lakey JR, Ryan EA, Korbutt GS, Toth E, Warnock GL, Kneteman NM, Rajotte RV: Islet transplantation in seven patients with type 1 diabetes mellitus using a glucocorticoid-free immunosuppressive regimen. N Engl J Med 2000;343:230–238.
49 Shapiro AM, Ricordi C, Hering BJ, Auchincloss H, Lindblad R, Robertson RP, Secchi A, Brendel MD, Berney T, Brennan DC, et al: International trial of the Edmonton protocol for islet transplantation. N Engl J Med 2006;355:1318–1330.
50 Phelps CJ, Koike C, Vaught TD, Boone J, Wells KD, Chen SH, Ball S, Specht SM, Polejaeva IA, Monahan JA, et al: Production of alpha 1,3-galactosyltransferase-deficient pigs. Science 2003;299:411–414.
51 Brazelton TR, Rossi FM, Keshet GI, Blau HM: From marrow to brain: expression of neuronal phenotypes in adult mice. Science 2000;290:1775–1779.
52 Ferrari G, Cusella-De Angelis G, Coletta M, Paolucci E, Stornaiuolo A, Cossu G, Mavilio F: Muscle regeneration by bone marrow-derived myogenic progenitors. Science 1998;279:1528–1530.
53 Krause DS, Theise ND, Collector MI, Henegariu O, Hwang S, Gardner R, Neutzel S, Sharkis SJ: Multi-organ, multi-lineage engraftment by a single bone marrow-derived stem cell. Cell 2001;105:369–377.
54 Lagasse E, Connors H, Al-Dhalimy M, Reitsma M, Dohse M, Osborne L, Wang X, Finegold M, Weissman IL, Grompe M: Purified hematopoietic stem cells can differentiate into hepatocytes in vivo. Nat Med 2000;6:1229–1234.
55 Mezey E, Chandross KJ, Harta G, Maki RA, McKercher SR: Turning blood into brain: cells bearing neuronal antigens generated in vivo from bone marrow. Science 2000;290:1779–1782.
56 Orlic D, Kajstura J, Chimenti S, Jakoniuk I, Anderson SM, Li B, Pickel J, McKay R, Nadal-Ginard B, Bodine DM, et al: Bone marrow cells regenerate infarcted myocardium. Nature 2001;410:701–705.
57 Petersen BE, Bowen WC, Patrene KD, Mars WM, Sullivan AK, Murase N, Boggs SS, Greenberger JS, Goff JP: Bone marrow as a potential source of hepatic oval cells. Science 1999;284:1168–1170.
58 Ianus A, Holz GG, Theise ND, Hussain MA: In vivo derivation of glucose-competent pancreatic endocrine cells from bone marrow without evidence of cell fusion. J Clin Invest 2003;111:843–850.
59 Lee VM, Stoffel M: Bone marrow: an extra-pancreatic hideout for the elusive pancreatic stem cell? J Clin Invest 2003;111:799–801.
60 Choi JB, Uchino H, Azuma K, Iwashita N, Tanaka Y, Mochizuki H, Migita M, Shimada T, Kawamori R, Watada H: Little evidence of transdifferentiation of bone marrow-derived cells into pancreatic beta cells. Diabetologia 2003;26:26.
61 Lechner A, Yang YG, Blacken RA, Wang L, Nolan AL, Habener JF: No evidence for significant transdifferentiation of bone marrow into pancreatic beta-cells in vivo. Diabetes 2004;53:616–623.
62 Taneera J, Rosengren A, Renstrom E, Nygren JM, Serup P, Rorsman P, Jacobsen SE: Failure of transplanted bone marrow cells to adopt a pancreatic beta-cell fate. Diabetes 2006;55:290–296.
63 Hess D, Li L, Martin M, Sakano S, Hill D, Strutt B, Thyssen S, Gray DA, Bhatia M: Bone marrow-derived stem cells initiate pancreatic regeneration. Nat Biotechnol 2003;21:763–770.
64 Lechner A, Habener JF: Bone marrow stem cells find a path to the pancreas. Nat Biotechnol 2003;21: 755–756.
65 Dor Y, Brown J, Martinez OI, Melton DA: Adult pancreatic beta-cells are formed by self-duplication rather than stem-cell differentiation. Nature 2004; 429:41–46.

66 Deutsch G, Jung J, Zheng M, Lora J, Zaret KS: A bipotential precursor population for pancreas and liver within the embryonic endoderm. Development 2001;128:871–881.
67 Ber I, Shternhall K, Perl S, Ohanuna Z, Goldberg I, Barshack I, Benvenisti-Zarum L, Meivar-Levy I, Ferber S: Functional, persistent, and extended liver to pancreas transdifferentiation. J Biol Chem 2003; 278:31950–31957.
68 Ferber S, Halkin A, Cohen H, Ber I, Einav Y, Goldberg I, Barshack I, Seijffers R, Kopolovic J, Kaiser N, Karasik A: Pancreatic and duodenal homeobox gene 1 induces expression of insulin genes in liver and ameliorates streptozotocin-induced hyperglycemia. Nat Med 2000;6:568–572.
69 Fodor A, Harel C, Fodor L, Armoni M, Salmon P, Trono D, Karnieli E: Adult rat liver cells transdifferentiated with lentiviral IPF1 vectors reverse diabetes in mice: an ex vivo gene therapy approach. Diabetologia 2007;50:121–130.
70 Horb ME, Shen CN, Tosh D, Slack JM: Experimental conversion of liver to pancreas. Curr Biol 2003; 13:105–115.
71 Kojima H, Fujimiya M, Matsumura K, Younan P, Imaeda H, Maeda M, Chan L: NeuroD-betacellulin gene therapy induces islet neogenesis in the liver and reverses diabetes in mice. Nat Med 2003;9:596–603.
72 Sapir T, Shternhall K, Meivar-Levy I, Blumenfeld T, Cohen H, Skutelsky E, Eventov-Friedman S, Barshack I, Goldberg I, Pri-Chen S, et al: Cell-replacement therapy for diabetes: generating functional insulin-producing tissue from adult human liver cells. Proc Natl Acad Sci USA 2005;102:7964–7969.
73 Zalzman M, Gupta S, Giri RK, Berkovich I, Sappal BS, Karnieli O, Zern MA, Fleischer N, Efrat S: Reversal of hyperglycemia in mice by using human expandable insulin-producing cells differentiated from fetal liver progenitor cells. Proc Natl Acad Sci USA 2003;100:7253–7258.
74 Soria B, Roche E, Berna G, Leon-Quinto T, Reig JA, Martin F: Insulin-secreting cells derived from embryonic stem cells normalize glycemia in streptozotocin-induced diabetic mice. Diabetes 2000;49: 157–162.
75 Lumelsky N, Blondel O, Laeng P, Velasco I, Ravin R, McKay R: Differentiation of embryonic stem cells to insulin-secreting structures similar to pancreatic islets. Science 2001;292:1389–1394.
76 Lendahl U, Zimmerman LB, McKay RD: CNS stem cells express a new class of intermediate filament protein. Cell 1990;60:585–595.
77 Zulewski H, Abraham EJ, Gerlach MJ, Daniel PB, Moritz W, Muller B, Vallejo M, Thomas MK, Habener JF: Multipotential nestin-positive stem cells isolated from adult pancreatic islets differentiate ex vivo into pancreatic endocrine, exocrine, and hepatic phenotypes. Diabetes 2001;50:521–533.
78 Delacour A, Nepote V, Trumpp A, Herrera PL: Nestin expression in pancreatic exocrine cell lineages. Mech Dev 2004;121:3–14.
79 Klein T, Ling Z, Heimberg H, Madsen OD, Heller RS, Serup P: Nestin is expressed in vascular endothelial cells in the adult human pancreas. J Histochem Cytochem 2003;51:697–706.
80 Lardon J, Rooman I, Bouwens L: Nestin expression in pancreatic stellate cells and angiogenic endothelial cells. Histochem Cell Biol 2002;117:535–540.
81 Selander L, Edlund H: Nestin is expressed in mesenchymal and non-epithelial cells of the developing mouse pancreas. Mech Dev 2002;113:189–192.
82 Hori Y, Rulifson IC, Tsai BC, Heit JJ, Cahoy JD, Kim SK: Growth inhibitors promote differentiation of insulin-producing tissue from embryonic stem cells. Proc Natl Acad Sci USA 2002;99:16105–16110.
83 Blyszczuk P, Czyz J, Kania G, Wagner M, Roll U, St-Onge L, Wobus AM: Expression of Pax4 in embryonic stem cells promotes differentiation of nestin-positive progenitor and insulin-producing cells. Proc Natl Acad Sci USA 2003;100:998–1003.
84 Sosa-Pineda B, Chowdhury K, Torres M, Oliver G, Gruss P: The Pax4 gene is essential for differentiation of insulin-producing β cells in the mammalian pancreas. Nature 1997;386:399–402.
85 Rajagopal J, Anderson WJ, Kume S, Martinez OI, Melton DA: Insulin staining of ES cell progeny from insulin uptake. Science 2003;299:363.
86 Hansson M, Tornning A, Frandsen U, Petri A, Rajagopal J, Englund MC, Heller RS, Hakansson J, Fleckner J, Skold HN, et al: Artifactual insulin release from differentiated embryonic stem cells. Diabetes 2004;53:2603–2609.
87 D'Amour KA, Bang AG, Eliazer S, Kelly OG, Agulnick AD, Smart NG, Moorman MA, Kroon E, Carpenter MK, Baetge EE: Production of pancreatic hormone-expressing endocrine cells from human embryonic stem cells. Nat Biotechnol 2006;24: 1392–1401.
88 D'Amour KA, Agulnick AD, Eliazer S, Kelly OG, Kroon E, Baetge EE: Efficient differentiation of human embryonic stem cells to definitive endoderm. Nat Biotechnol 2005;23:1534–1541.

Dr. Raphael Scharfmann
Hôpital Necker, INSERM U845, Faculty Necker, 156, rue de Vaugirard, FR–75730 Paris (France)
Tel. +33 140 61 5565, Fax +33 143 06 0443, E-Mail scharfmann@necker.fr

Shield JPH, Scharfmann R (eds): Development of the Pancreas and Neonatal Diabetes.
Endocr Dev. Basel, Karger, 2007, vol 12, pp 12–23

Overview of Neonatal Diabetes

Julian P. Hamilton-Shield

University of Bristol and Bristol Royal Hospital for Children, Bristol, UK

Abstract

Diabetes developing within the first 6 months of life is rarely, if ever, caused by a classic type 1 diabetes-related autoimmune process. Currently, patients developing diabetes before 6 months of age are defined as having neonatal diabetes although this terminology possibly needs amending. Neonatal diabetes has a transient and permanent form and over 10 distinct genetic anomalies or mutations have been identified causing the disease. Transient neonatal diabetes can be caused by defects in the normal methylation pattern of an imprinted gene on chromosome 6 and by mutations in the 2 genes encoding the β-cell ATP-sensitive potassium channel which is vital to normal glucose-stimulated insulin secretion. A genetic cause can be identified in over 90% of transient cases. Permanent neonatal diabetes can be caused by mutations in β-cell transcription factors leading to abnormal pancreatic development often with other significant developmental anomalies, by defects in the glucose sensing, insulin secretory network and by accelerated β-cell destruction. About 30% of cases of permanent diabetes have yet to have a genetic cause identified.

In 1993, Prof. David Baum and I published a letter in the *Lancet* relating the story of a child who had diabetes as a baby that resolved only to come back in adolescence [1]. We suggested at the time that this condition termed 'neonatal diabetes' might be informative to our broader understanding of pancreas development and the pathogenesis of diabetes. Since then research has revealed at least 10 genes involved in disease causation and in many children, our understanding of the underlying cause has revolutionized therapeutic options and improved genetic counselling. Although the term 'neonatal diabetes' is a misnomer as the various conditions can present up to 6 months of age and the neonatal period is strictly the first month of life, the term will be used throughout this article for ease of terminology.

Neonatal diabetes can be simply subdivided into transient (TNDM) and permanent (PNDM) types based on whether the diabetes resolves in infancy or continues throughout life. In reality, virtually all if not all children presenting with diabetes before 6 months of life will have a monogenic cause for their diabetes with classic autoimmune type 1 diabetes being restricted to children presenting with diabetes after that age [2, 3]. Although not universally so, the vast majority of children born with neonatal diabetes syndromes are quite severely growth-retarded, reflecting the importance of normal insulin secretion for third-trimester fetal growth.

In this chapter, I will briefly describe each of the known monogenic causes of neonatal diabetes, splitting the group into transient and permanent causes and then describing conditions in terms of the putative pathology in each condition.

Transient Neonatal Diabetes

Chromosome 6q Anomalies (OMIM 601410)

Transient diabetes in infancy that resolves within the first 3 months of life is a well-recognized phenomenon. Clinically these children are born after significant intrauterine growth retardation, developing diabetes at a mean age of 3 days. The diabetes is characterized by severe hyperglycaemia and dehydration but little or no ketosis [4]. This condition remains the most frequent single cause of neonatal diabetes and the most frequent cause of the transient form (approx. 70%) [5].

In 1995, we identified 2 patients with paternal uniparental (iso)disomy of chromosome 6q24 causing transient neonatal diabetes [6]. Effectively, the child inherits two copies of the same chromosome 6 from the father with no contribution from the mother. The process of uniparental (iso)disomy can uncover autosomal recessive conditions as the child can inherit two copies of a single mutation of a recessive gene carried on one of the parent of origin's chromosomes or it can imply that a gene or genes are imprinted, whereby the parent of origin affects a gene's functional phenotype. In simple terms, imprinted genes are switched off by the addition of a methyl group(s) generally in the promoter region, preventing gene transcription which can either be on the maternal or paternal copy of a gene. 6q anomalies are due to disorders of imprinting. Two copies of paternal chromosome 6, an unbalanced duplication (extra copy) of paternal 6q24 [7, 8] or loss of imprinting (loss of methylation) from maternal 6q24 all cause TNDM [9] due to overexpression of gene(s) within the TNDM locus.

Interestingly, we have recently been able to demonstrate that children with TNDM due specifically to a loss of maternal methylation at the TNDM locus actually display a spectrum of reduced maternal methylation at other imprinted loci. This probably accounts for some of the associated features of TNDM and 6q anomalies such as macroglossia and anterior abdominal wall defects, classically associated with Beckwith-Wiedemann syndrome relating to loss of methylation at *KvDMR* [10, 11].

There are two potential imprinted genes responsible for TNDM at the 6q locus: *ZAC* and/or *HYMAI*. We recently developed an overexpressing mouse model of the TNDM locus. This mouse displays many of the phenotypic features of 6q anomalies although birth weight was normal. We have shown that TNDM overexpression reduces the expression of the key transcription factor *IPF1* in the embryonic pancreas of these mice [12]. At the American Diabetes Association meeting in 2006, Polychronakos and Xiaoyu [13] presented data on specific and controlled *ZAC* overexpression on β-cell function in the INS1 rat β-cell line, demonstrating that it was likely to be the gene responsible for TNDM in 6q anomalies. *ZAC* is a zinc finger protein which regulates apoptosis and cell cycle arrest through DNA binding and transactivation [14]. Recently, it has been demonstrated that a major target for *ZAC* is the peroxisome proliferator-activated receptor γ *(PPARγ)* that is up-regulated by direct *ZAC* binding to the proximal *PPARγ* 1 promoter [15]. *PPARγ* activation, which would be expected with *ZAC* overexpression, causes inhibition of β-cell proliferation whilst also compromising glucose-stimulated insulin secretion [16, 17].

All children with 6q anomalies have been associated with a transient form of diabetes in infancy, but this has been reported to relapse around the time of adolescence in a majority, although there probably is an element of reporting bias in the quoted levels of around 60% [4]. Interestingly, although the relapse is characterized by a loss of the classic insulin response to hyperglycaemia, we have some evidence that insulin is still available, as an excellent insulin secretory response has been documented on glucagon stimulation suggesting that the G-coupled protein receptor response remains intact through increasing cAMP and perhaps might be an area of therapeutic intervention in the future [18].

The Islet K_{ATP} Channel

This channel is a critical regulator of β-cell insulin secretion. In the normal response to increased glucose exposure and its metabolism within the β-cell, ATP levels increase with a concomitant decrease in Mg-ADP, allowing closure of the K_{ATP} channel and membrane depolarization, permitting calcium influx into the cell, which leads to insulin secretion. The K_{ATP} channel is a hetero-octamer made up of two subunits encoded by the *KCNJ11* and *ABCC8* genes. In neonatal diabetes caused by mutations in the *KCNJ11* gene, the channel is variably unresponsive to increased ATP levels making the membrane hyperpolarized, preventing influx of calcium and efflux of insulin [5]. In the case of ABCC8 mutations, the basal Mg-nucleotide-dependent stimulatory action of SUR1, encoded by ABCC8, is increased, which effectively prevents closure.

KCNJ11 Transient Neonatal Diabetes (OMIM 610582)

In 2005, Yorifuji et al. [19] reported a 4-generation family with dominantly inherited diabetes mellitus observed in 3 generations due to a cys42-to-arg mutation in the *KCNJ11* gene. None of the patients in this family had permanent neonatal diabetes.

The proband had transient neonatal diabetes, and his paternal grandfather had been diagnosed with diabetes at 3 years of age. The proband's paternal aunt developed gestational diabetes at age 26, which was transient, but she was diagnosed with adult-onset diabetes at age 28. The proband's father developed diabetes at age 22. Further reports have confirmed that mutations in this gene can cause transient neonatal diabetes and apparently familial diabetes without a history of neonatal problems in all generations [20]. This form of neonatal diabetes is likely to relapse in later life [21].

ABCC8 Transient Neonatal Diabetes (OMIM 610374)

In 2006, Babenko et al. [22] reported that heterozygous mutations in the gene *ABCC8* can cause transient neonatal diabetes although some cases had a permanent form responsive to sulphonylureas. In at least one example, a child with the transient form has relapsed in later life, the diabetes being found responsive to treatment with sulphonylurea therapy [23].

KCNJ11 and *ABCC8* mutations make up the majority of those patients with TNDM who do not have a 6q anomaly. The intra-uterine growth retardation is not so profound as in 6q anomalies (mean birth weight 2,570 vs. 1,950 g) whilst the age of presentation is also later (4 vs. 0 weeks) as is the time to remission (35 vs. 13 weeks) [21].

Permanent Neonatal Diabetes

Defects in β-Cell Transcription Genes

Insulin Promoter Factor 1 Deficiency (OMIM 260370)

In 1997, Doris Stoffers et al. [24] described a child with permanent neonatal diabetes and pancreatic exocrine insufficiency due to pancreatic agenesis. The proband was homozygous for a mutation (Pro63fsdelC) in *IPF1,* a gene involved in the master control of exocrine and endocrine pancreatic development, being responsible for the coordinated development of the pancreas in utero as well as for the continued functional integrity of pancreatic β-islet cells. Within the extended family were 8 individuals in 6 generations with early-onset diabetes akin to type 2 diabetes. These were identified as heterozygotes for the same mutation with the mutant truncated isoform of *IPF1* acting as a dominant negative inhibitor of wild-type *IPF1* activity. The illness resulting from heterozygosity was reassigned as maturity-onset diabetes of the young type 4 [25]. Additional studies have also identified that less severe *IPF1* mutations can cause autosomal dominant late-onset forms of type 2 diabetes that account for around 6% of a French cohort of multiplex type 2 diabetic families [26]. Only one further case report of pancreatic agenesis has been ascribed to an *IPF1* mutation and this was a compound heterozygous mutation of the gene [27]. Due to the complete absence of pancreatic tissue, exocrine function is also severely compromised requiring the use of pancreatic enzyme supplementation for normal growth.

GLIS Family Zinc Finger Protein 3 (OMIM 610192)
In June 2006, Senee et al. [28] described a frameshift mutation or deletions in the transcription factor *GLIS3* in 3 consanguineous families with a history of neonatal diabetes, congenital hypothyroidism and facial dysmorphology (large, flat, square-shaped face with a thin and bird-shaped curved nose). Additional features seen in some, but not all patients included congenital glaucoma, liver fibrosis and cystic kidneys [28]. *GLIS3* belongs to the GLIS subfamily of Kruppel-like zinc finger proteins and functions as an activator and repressor of transcription [29]. Fifty percent of the children so far identified with this condition have died before their 2nd birthday.

Permanent Neonatal Diabetes with Cerebellar Hypoplasia (OMIM 609069)
In 1999, a group identified a new recessively inherited disease of neonatal diabetes associated with cerebellar hypoplasia [30]. The 3 children of consanguineous, Pakistani origin had dysmorphic features (low-set ears, triangular facies, talipes equinovarus and joint stiffness), associated with neonatal diabetes, microcephaly, recurrent apnoeic attacks and absent cerebellar tissue on brain imaging (fig. 1). A further child of North European descent was later identified with an identical phenotype in whom an autopsy demonstrated complete pancreatic agenesis. Further studies on this child and the original family led to the identification of the gene responsible, *PTF1A*. This gene encodes the pancreas transcription factor 1α which is essential for normal pancreatic and cerebellar development [31]. In the pancreas, development begins with the formation of buds at specific sites in the embryonic foregut endoderm with *PTF1A* being expressed at these early stages in the progenitors of pancreatic ducts, exocrine and endocrine cells. So far, all children described with this condition have died in infancy, not from diabetes but associated respiratory failure probably secondary to the brain anomalies.

Hepatic Nuclear Factor 1β
In humans, it has been shown that heterozygous mutations of the HNF1β gene *(TCF2)* are associated with a form of maturity-onset diabetes of the young (type 5), which is characterized by dominantly inherited diabetes mellitus associated with renal cysts. Early expression of *TCF2* is seen in the kidney, liver, bile ducts, thymus, genital tract, pancreas, lung, and gut. In 1 family, a missense heterozygous mutation of HNF1β was associated with neonatal diabetes and some small cysts in 1 child but only transient hyperglycaemia with more profound renal dysplasia in the other sibling [32]. The child with 'neonatal diabetes' was receiving total parenteral nutrition which can cause iatrogenic hyperglycaemia in neonates and whether this will turn out to truly represent a cause for neonatal diabetes is still, I believe, open to question.

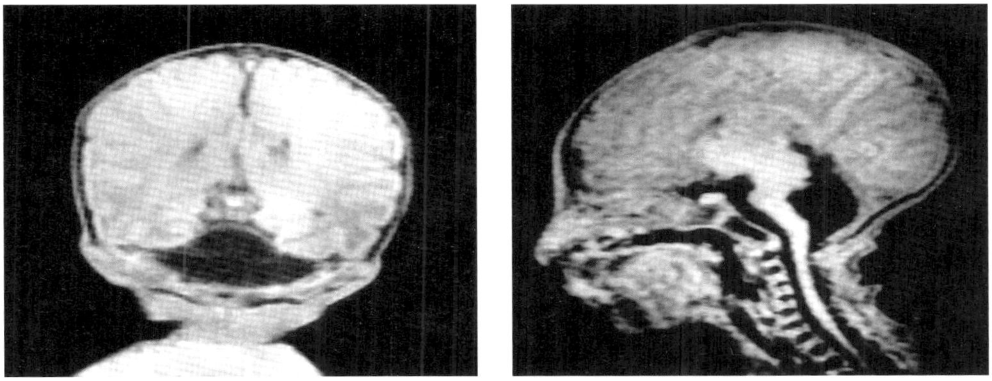

Fig. 1. Demonstrating cerebellar hypoplasia/aplasia in one of the original cases caused by PTFA1 mutation and described by the author. Taken from Hoveyda et al. [30].

Defects in β-Cell Function

KCNJ11 Permanent Neonatal Diabetes (OMIM 600937)

The second most common cause of neonatal diabetes and the most common cause of the permanent form is that induced by heterozygous activating mutations in the *KCNJ11* gene, which encodes the Kir6.2 subunit of the K_{ATP} channel, a critical regulator of β-cell insulin secretion [33]. Although the majority has been identified to cause permanent neonatal diabetes, a few have been associated with a transient condition akin to that caused by 6q anomalies [20]. In normal circumstances, the K_{ATP} channel closes in response to increased intracellular ATP induced by glucose metabolism in the islet cell. In diabetes, due to mutations in this gene, the channel displays decreased sensitivity to ATP and the β-cells remain hyperpolarized and unable to secrete insulin [34].

The babies are born small for gestational age, but not as small as in some other neonatal diabetes conditions [mean birth weight: 2,497 g (SD 690) vs. 1,987 g (SD 510) in babies with 6q anomalies] [5]. Thirty percent have ketoacidosis and all display low insulin levels in the face of quite dramatic hyperglycaemia. The median age of presentation is around 3–4 weeks of age as opposed to 6q anomalies that tend to present in the 1st week of life although the spectrum in both conditions is such that birth weight or the age of presentation cannot be used to distinguish between the two conditions. About 20% have associated neurological disease with developmental delay and sometimes epilepsy or muscle weakness, reflecting a role for the same potassium channel in the central nervous system. The most severe end of this spectrum has been entitled 'DEND' (developmental delay, epilepsy and neonatal diabetes) in which children can be severely affected. There is also an intermediate condition (i-DEND) with milder developmental delay and no epilepsy. The mutations causing isolated diabetes produce less change in ATP sensitivity than those associated with diabetes and neurological disease (Q52R, V59G) [35].

Sulphonylureas, a class of drugs often used in type 2 diabetes, close K_{ATP} channels by an ATP-independent mechanism. An increasing number of patients with this condition have successfully transferred to oral sulphonylurea therapy needing a dose of between 0.5 and 1.0 mg/kg/day of glibenclamide [36, 37], a relatively large dose compared to that used in adults with type 2 diabetes. A recent paper demonstrated that 90% (n = 44/49; ages 3 months to 36 years) can be successfully transferred to oral therapy with a highly significant and sustained improvement in glycated haemoglobin (from 8.1 to 6.4%). Although a successful switch to sulphonylureas is not mutation specific, it appears that those with neurological features are less likely to be successful [38]. The author currently has 3 patients on therapy with Kir6.2 mutations all of whom responded to sulphonylurea therapy and all with glycated haemoglobin levels around the 6% level indicating good glycaemic control with no significant history of hypoglycaemia.

ABCC8 Mutation Permanent Neonatal Diabetes (OMIM 600509)

The experience of the French group who originally described *ABCC8* mutations was that a significant majority caused transient neonatal diabetes with far fewer permanent cases [23]. However, a recent publication from the UK demonstrates that mutations in the *ABCC8* gene encoding the SUR1 subunit accounted for 27% of non-Kir6.2 PNDM in their cohort. Furthermore, not only did they identify heterozygous activating mutations but also homozygous, autosomal recessive disease and that caused by compound activating/inactivating mutations [39]. The response to sulphonylureas in those permanent cases with heterozygous mutations has been very encouraging [22], although the author has not been able to transfer treatment from insulin to a sulphonylurea in 1 homozygous, recessive case, perhaps because 'homozygous' islet cells for mutant *ABCC8* channels are more adversely affected than those displaying a mixture of mutant and wild-type SUR1 [22].

Homozygous Glucokinase Mutations (OMIM 138079)

Glucokinase is responsible for the first step in glucose metabolism within the islet cell and as such acts as a 'sensor' controlling insulin secretion. Heterozygous inactivating mutations in glucokinase cause maturity-onset diabetes of the young type 2, characterized by mild hyperglycaemia, which is present at birth, but is often only detected later in life and is rarely, if ever, associated with diabetes complications. However, infants born to parents both heterozygous for inactivating mutations in glucokinase can be rendered homozygous without any glycolytic activity at all and profound neonatal diabetes [40]. Diabetes usually presents in the first week of life with moderate to severe intra-uterine growth retardation (1.5–2 kg) [41]. Perhaps not unexpectedly, there is often a degree of consanguinity. Clinicians should look for a history of maternal gestational diabetes which should prompt testing for fasting glucose levels in both parents. If both parents have mild glucose intolerance, a screen for glucokinase mutations is then warranted.

Neonatal Diabetes due to β-Cell Destruction

Immune Dysregulation, Polyendocrinopathy, Enteropathy, X-Linked Syndrome (FOXP3 and CD25 Mutations) (OMIM 304790)

The scurfy mouse is a natural mutant clinically resembling human immune dysregulation, polyendocrinopathy, enteropathy, X-linked syndrome (IPEX). Displaying an X-linked recessive pattern of inheritance, the disease causes runting, ichthyosis, progressive anaemia, thrombocytopaenia, hypogonadism in males, increased infections and diarrhoea with death by 3–4 weeks of age [42]. The disease is due to a mutation in the *Foxp3* gene encoding for a protein called 'scurfin' which is essential for normal immune homeostasis with scurfy T cells being hyperresponsive to activation and resistant to cyclosporin. In 2001, the human disease was also identified as due to mutations in *FOXP3* [43]. Entitled 'immune dysregulation, polyendocrinopathy, enteropathy, X-linked syndrome', its major features are early-onset diabetes (often neonatal) and diarrhoea with small intestinal pathology such as villous atrophy and inflammatory infiltrate. The condition is probably the only one described in children developing diabetes under the age of 6 months in which autoimmunity plays a part. Type 1 diabetes auto-antibodies (GAD, IAA, ICA) are frequently described as are those directed against the thyroid gland and various other organs [44]. Other features frequently described in the human condition other than diabetes, enteropathy and severe failure to thrive include eczema, haemolytic anaemia, thrombocytopaenia and hypothyroidism. Enteropathy (100%), failure to thrive (>90%) and diabetes (>90%) occur in almost all cases [45]. The autoimmunity is extremely aggressive and destructive. Given that immune dysregulation appears to underlie this condition the most obvious routes for treatment have been applied with varying degrees of success. Immunosuppression with cyclosporin or tacrolimus has proved of limited value in general although some patients have responded better than others [44]. The immunosuppression has often been at the cost of significant medication toxicity to other organs such as the kidneys [46]. An alternative approach of bone marrow transplantation seems to offer most hope of cure. Early results in at least 4 cases showed fairly promising effects in the short term on diarrhoea, weight gain and possibly diabetes but 3 patients subsequently succumbed to infection often with evidence of an accompanying lymphoproliferative disorder [44, 47]. A fourth patient did not have diabetes nor a mutation in the coding region of *FOXP3* but did have a deletion in the promoter upstream of the gene and reduced levels of *FOXP3* mRNA. This child remains well 16 months after transplantation with complete clinical and immunological remission [48]. Recently, a new strategy for bone marrow transplantation has been adopted with reduced intensity conditioning using alemtuzumab, fludarabine and melphalan [49]. The 4 children on whom this has been tried remain alive although late complications are still problematic.

Importantly, approximately 1/3 of patients with the IPEX syndrome do not have mutations in *FOXP3*. Very recently, a patient has been identified with a *CD25* mutation (interleukin 2 receptor α), also causing an IPEX-like picture and in cases with normal *FOXP3* screening studies should extend to examining *CD25* [50].

Wolcott-Rallison Syndrome (OMIM 226980)
This is an autosomal recessive disorder characterized by infancy-onset (often within the neonatal period) diabetes associated with a spondylo-epiphyseal dysplasia. In addition, there is a constellation of other features such as hepatomegaly and hepatic dysfunction/failure, mental retardation, renal failure and early death in many cases although some children are alive aged 10 years and evidence of heterogeneity in phenotype even within families is described [51–53]. In 2000, Delepine et al. [54] used 2 consanguineous families to map the condition to the locus 2p12. Within this locus lay the gene *EIF2AK3* that is highly expressed in islet cells acting as a regulator of protein synthesis. Proteins and insulin are manufactured in the endoplasmic reticulum. In response to environmental stresses, cells down-regulate protein synthesis by phosphorylation of the α-subunit of eukaryotic translation initiation factor 2 by eukaryotic translation initiation factor 2 kinase 3. Malfolded proteins in the endoplasmic reticulum inhibit further translation initiation mediated by increased phosphorylation of the α-subunit of eukaryotic translation initiation factor 2. A targeted mutation of the mouse gene *Eif2ak3* (PERK) led to an accumulation of malfolded proteins in the endoplasmic reticulum with resultant abnormally elevated protein synthesis and increased stress on the endoplasmic reticulum folding machinery [55]. PERK is highly expressed in the mouse pancreas. The PERK knockout mouse demonstrates normal pancreatic endocrine and exocrine development. However, postnatally it develops endoplasmic reticulum distension accompanied by increased cell death and progressive diabetes mellitus and pancreatic exocrine failure [56]. Further analysis within the consanguineous Wolcott-Rallison families confirmed frameshift or amino acid substitution mutations occurring in *EIF2AK3* segregating with the disorder in each family [54].

Conclusions

The most frequent cause of transient neonatal diabetes are 6q anomalies with the majority of the remaining cases accounted for by mutations in *KCJN11* or *ABCC8*. Whilst diabetes in these children goes into remission, there is good evidence in all examples that there is a significant likelihood of relapse in later life possibly related to times of metabolic stress such as puberty or during intercurrent infections. In approximately 70% of cases of permanent neonatal diabetes, a genetic cause can now be identified. *KCJN11* heterozygous activating mutations are the most frequent cause, accounting for around 30% of all cases with *ABCC8* cases making up a further 15%. These two channelopathies are remarkable given their likelihood to respond to oral sulphonylureas rather than requiring lifelong insulin therapy. Two conditions causing β-cell destruction make up a further 20% of reported cases, *FOXP3* and *CD25* mutations through autoimmune destruction of islet cells and *EIF2AK3* through endoplasmic reticulum stress and β-cell failure. These conditions are potentially difficult to manage and associated with a high level of early morbidity and mortality. Mutations in β-cell transcription genes make up a further 5% of permanent cases. Around 30% of permanent neonatal diabetes cases remain unsolved in terms of the underlying genetic basis. Identifying the mechanisms of pathology will undoubtedly further our understanding of pancreatic development and function. One final observation is that the incidence of neonatal diabetes appears to be increasing or at least its recognition as a distinct clinical entity is increasing. In a survey conducted in the British Isles last year on the incidence of non-type 1 diabetes in childhood, neonatal diabetes was notified as the most frequent recognized cause of syndromic diabetes with 9 cases being notified during the year-long study period [57].

References

1 Shield JP, Baum JD: Is transient neonatal diabetes a risk factor for diabetes in later life? Lancet 1993;341:693.

2 Iafusco D, Stazi MA, Cotichini R, Cotellessa M, Martinucci ME, Mazzella M, et al: Permanent diabetes mellitus in the first year of life. Diabetologia 2002;45:798–804.

3 Edghill EL, Dix RJ, Flanagan SE, Bingley PJ, Hattersley AT, Ellard S, et al: HLA genotyping supports a nonautoimmune etiology in patients diagnosed with diabetes under the age of 6 months. Diabetes 2006;55:1895–1898.

4 Temple IK, Gardner RJ, Mackay DJ, Barber JC, Robinson DO, Shield JP: Transient neonatal diabetes: widening the understanding of the etiopathogenesis of diabetes. Diabetes 2000;49:1359–1366.

5 Slingerland AS, Hattersley AT: Mutations in the Kir6.2 subunit of the K_{ATP} channel and permanent neonatal diabetes: new insights and new treatment. Ann Med 2005;37:186–195.

6 Temple IK, James RS, Crolla JA, Sitch FL, Jacobs PA, Howell WM, et al: An imprinted gene(s) for diabetes? Nat Genet 1995;9:110–112.

7 Temple IK, Gardner RJ, Robinson DO, Kibirige MS, Ferguson AW, Baum JD, et al: Further evidence for an imprinted gene for neonatal diabetes localised to chromosome 6q22–q23. Hum Mol Genet 1996;5:1117–1121.

8 Cave H, Polak M, Drunat S, Denamur E, Czernichow P: Refinement of the 6q chromosomal region implicated in transient neonatal diabetes. Diabetes 2000;49:108–113.

9 Gardner RJ, Mackay DJ, Mungall AJ, Polychronakos C, Siebert R, Shield JP, et al: An imprinted locus associated with transient neonatal diabetes mellitus. Hum Mol Genet 2000;9:589–596.

10 Mackay DJ, Hahnemann JM, Boonen SE, Poerksen S, Bunyan DJ, White HE, et al: Epimutation of the TNDM locus and the Beckwith-Wiedemann syndrome centromeric locus in individuals with transient neonatal diabetes mellitus. Hum Genet 2006;119:179–184.

11 Mackay DJ, Boonen SE, Clayton-Smith J, Goodship J, Hahnemann JM, Kant SG, et al: A maternal hypomethylation syndrome presenting as transient neonatal diabetes mellitus. Hum Genet 2006;120:262–269.

12 Ma D, Shield JP, Dean W, Leclerc I, Knauf C, Burcelin RR, et al: Impaired glucose homeostasis in transgenic mice expressing the human transient neonatal diabetes mellitus locus, TNDM. J Clin Invest 2004;114:339–348.

13 Polychronakos C, Xiaoyu D: Graded Overexpression of ZAC Impairs Glucose Stimulated Insulin Secretion in Beta-Cells. Washington, American Diabetes Association, 2006.

14 Spengler D, Villalba M, Hoffmann A, Pantaloni C, Houssami S, Bockaert J, et al: Regulation of apoptosis and cell cycle arrest by Zac1, a novel zinc finger protein expressed in the pituitary gland and the brain. EMBO J 1997;16:2814–2825.

15 Barz T, Hoffmann A, Panhuysen M, Spengler D: Peroxisome proliferator-activated receptor gamma is a Zac target gene mediating Zac antiproliferation. Cancer Res 2006;66:11975–11982.

16 Rosen ED, Kulkarni RN, Sarraf P, Ozcan U, Okada T, Hsu CH, et al: Targeted elimination of peroxisome proliferator-activated receptor gamma in beta cells leads to abnormalities in islet mass without compromising glucose homeostasis. Mol Cell Biol 2003;23:7222–7229.

17 Ravnskjaer K, Boergesen M, Rubi B, Larsen JK, Nielsen T, Fridriksson J, et al: Peroxisome proliferator-activated receptor alpha (PPARalpha) potentiates, whereas PPARgamma attenuates, glucose-stimulated insulin secretion in pancreatic beta-cells. Endocrinology 2005;146:3266–3276.

18 Valerio G, Franzese A, Salerno M, Muzzi G, Cecere G, Temple KI, et al: Beta-cell dysfunction in classic transient neonatal diabetes is characterized by impaired insulin response to glucose but normal response to glucagon. Diabetes Care 2004;27:2405–2408.

19 Yorifuji T, Nagashima K, Kurokawa K, Kawai M, Oishi M, Akazawa Y, et al: The C42R mutation in the Kir6.2 (KCNJ11) gene as a cause of transient neonatal diabetes, childhood diabetes, or later-onset, apparently type 2 diabetes mellitus. J Clin Endocrinol Metab 2005;90:3174–3178.

20 Gloyn AL, Reimann F, Girard C, Edghill EL, Proks P, Pearson ER, et al: Relapsing diabetes can result from moderately activating mutations in KCNJ11. Hum Mol Genet 2005;14:925–934.

21 Flanagan SE, Patch AM, Mackay DJG, Edghill EL, Gloyn AL, Robinson D, et al: Mutations in ATP-sensitive K^+ channel genes cause transient neonatal diabetes and permanent diabetes in childhood or adulthood. Diabetes 2007;56:1930–1937.

22 Babenko AP, Polak M, Cave H, Busiah K, Czernichow P, Scharfmann R, et al: Activating mutations in the ABCC8 gene in neonatal diabetes mellitus. N Engl J Med 2006;355:456–466.

23 Vaxillaire M, Dechaume A, Busiah K, Cave H, Pereira S, Scharfmann R, et al: New ABCC8 mutations in relapsing neonatal diabetes and clinical features. Diabetes 2007;56:1737–1741.

24 Stoffers DA, Zinkin NT, Stanojevic V, Clarke WL, Habener JF: Pancreatic agenesis attributable to a single nucleotide deletion in the human IPF1 gene coding sequence. Nat Genet 1997;15:106–110.

25 Stoffers DA, Stanojevic V, Habener JF: Insulin promoter factor-1 gene mutation linked to early-onset type 2 diabetes mellitus directs expression of a dominant negative isoprotein. J Clin Invest 1998; 102:232–241.

26 Hani EH, Stoffers DA, Chevre JC, Durand E, Stanojevic V, Dina C, et al: Defective mutations in the insulin promoter factor-1 (IPF-1) gene in late-onset type 2 diabetes mellitus. J Clin Invest 1999;104: R41–R48.

27 Schwitzgebel VM, Mamin A, Brun T, Ritz-Laser B, Zaiko M, Maret A, et al: Agenesis of human pancreas due to decreased half-life of insulin promoter factor 1. J Clin Endocrinol Metab 2003;88:4398–4406.

28 Senee V, Chelala C, Duchatelet S, Feng D, Blanc H, Cossec JC, et al: Mutations in GLIS3 are responsible for a rare syndrome with neonatal diabetes mellitus and congenital hypothyroidism. Nat Genet 2006; 38:682–687.

29 Kim YS, Nakanishi G, Lewandoski M, Jetten AM: GLIS3, a novel member of the GLIS subfamily of Kruppel-like zinc finger proteins with repressor and activation functions. Nucleic Acids Res 2003; 31:5513–5525.

30 Hoveyda N, Shield JP, Garrett C, Chong WK, Beardsall K, Bentsi-Enchill E, et al: Neonatal diabetes mellitus and cerebellar hypoplasia/agenesis: report of a new recessive syndrome. J Med Genet 1999;36:700–704.

31 Sellick GS, Barker KT, Stolte-Dijkstra I, Fleischmann C, Coleman RJ, Garrett C, et al: Mutations in PTF1A cause pancreatic and cerebellar agenesis. Nat Genet 2004;36:1301–1305.

32 Yorifuji T, Kurokawa K, Mamada M, Imai T, Kawai M, Nishi Y, et al: Neonatal diabetes mellitus and neonatal polycystic, dysplastic kidneys: phenotypically discordant recurrence of a mutation in the hepatocyte nuclear factor-1beta gene due to germline mosaicism. J Clin Endocrinol Metab 2004;89:2905–2908.

33 Gloyn AL, Pearson ER, Antcliff JF, Proks P, Bruining GJ, Slingerland AS, et al: Activating mutations in the gene encoding the ATP-sensitive potassium-channel subunit Kir6.2 and permanent neonatal diabetes. N Engl J Med 2004;350:1838–1849.

34 Hattersley AT, Ashcroft FM: Activating mutations in Kir6.2 and neonatal diabetes: new clinical syndromes, new scientific insights, and new therapy. Diabetes 2005;54:2503–2513.

35 Proks P, Antcliff JF, Lippiat J, Gloyn AL, Hattersley AT, Ashcroft FM: Molecular basis of Kir6.2 mutations associated with neonatal diabetes or neonatal diabetes plus neurological features. Proc Natl Acad Sci USA 2004;101:17539–17544.

36 Sagen JV, Raeder H, Hathout E, Shehadeh N, Gudmundsson K, Baevre H, et al: Permanent neonatal diabetes due to mutations in KCNJ11 encoding Kir6.2: patient characteristics and initial response to sulfonylurea therapy. Diabetes 2004;53:2713–2718.

37 Klupa T, Edghill EL, Nazim J, Sieradzki J, Ellard S, Hattersley AT, et al: The identification of a R201H mutation in KCNJ11, which encodes Kir6.2, and successful transfer to sustained-release sulphonylurea therapy in a subject with neonatal diabetes: evidence for heterogeneity of beta cell function among carriers of the R201H mutation. Diabetologia 2005;48:1029–1031.

38 Pearson ER, Flechtner I, Njolstad PR, Malecki MT, Flanagan SE, Larkin B, et al: Switching from insulin to oral sulfonylureas in patients with diabetes due to Kir6.2 mutations. N Engl J Med 2006;355:457–477.
39 Ellard S, Flanagan SE, Patch AM, Harries LW, Parrish A, Edghill EL, et al: Activating and inactivating SUR1 mutations in patients with neonatal diabetes. Am J Med Genet, in press.
40 Njolstad PR, Sovik O, Cuesta-Munoz A, Bjorkhaug L, Massa O, Barbetti F, et al: Neonatal diabetes mellitus due to complete glucokinase deficiency. N Engl J Med 2001;344:1588–1592.
41 Njolstad PR, Sagen JV, Bjorkhaug L, Odili S, Shehadeh N, Bakry D, et al: Permanent neonatal diabetes caused by glucokinase deficiency: inborn error of the glucose-insulin signaling pathway. Diabetes 2003;52:2854–2860.
42 Brunkow ME, Jeffery EW, Hjerrild KA, Paeper B, Clark LB, Yasayko SA, et al: Disruption of a new forkhead/winged-helix protein, scurfin, results in the fatal lymphoproliferative disorder of the scurfy mouse. Nat Genet 2001;27:68–73.
43 Wildin RS, Ramsdell F, Peake J, Faravelli F, Casanova JL, Buist N, et al: X-linked neonatal diabetes mellitus, enteropathy and endocrinopathy syndrome is the human equivalent of mouse scurfy. Nat Genet 2001;27:18–20.
44 Wildin RS, Smyk-Pearson S, Filipovich AH: Clinical and molecular features of the immunodysregulation, polyendocrinopathy, enteropathy, X linked (IPEX) syndrome. J Med Genet 2002;39:537–545.
45 Gambineri E, Torgerson TR, Ochs HD: Immune dysregulation, polyendocrinopathy, enteropathy, and X-linked inheritance (IPEX), a syndrome of systemic autoimmunity caused by mutations of FOXP3, a critical regulator of T-cell homeostasis. Curr Opin Rheumatol 2003;15:430–435.
46 Ruemmele FM, Brousse N, Goulet O: Autoimmune enteropathy: molecular concepts. Curr Opin Gastroenterol 2004;20:587–591.
47 Baud O, Goulet O, Canioni D, Le Deist F, Radford I, Rieu D, et al: Treatment of the immune dysregulation, polyendocrinopathy, enteropathy, X-linked syndrome (IPEX) by allogeneic bone marrow transplantation. N Engl J Med 2001;344:1758–1762.
48 Mazzolari E, Forino C, Fontana M, D'Ippolito C, Lanfranchi A, Gambineri E, et al: A new case of IPEX receiving bone marrow transplantation. Bone Marrow Transplant 2005;35:1033–1034.
49 Rao A, Kamani N, Filipovich A, Lee SM, Davies SM, Dalal J, et al: Successful bone marrow transplantation for IPEX syndrome after reduced-intensity conditioning. Blood 2007;109:383–385.
50 Caudy AA, Reddy ST, Chatila T, Atkinson JP, Verbsky JW: CD25 deficiency causes an immune dysregulation, polyendocrinopathy, enteropathy, X-linked-like syndrome, and defective IL-10 expression from CD4 lymphocytes. J Allergy Clin Immunol 2007;119:482–487.
51 Senee V, Vattem KM, Delepine M, Rainbow LA, Haton C, Lecoq A, et al: Wolcott-Rallison Syndrome: clinical, genetic, and functional study of EIF2AK3 mutations and suggestion of genetic heterogeneity. Diabetes 2004;53:1876–1883.
52 Durocher F, Faure R, Labrie Y, Pelletier L, Bouchard I, Laframboise R: A novel mutation in the EIF2AK3 gene with variable expressivity in two patients with Wolcott-Rallison syndrome. Clin Genet 2006;70:34–38.
53 Iyer S, Korada M, Rainbow L, Kirk J, Brown RM, Shaw N, et al: Wolcott-Rallison syndrome: a clinical and genetic study of three children, novel mutation in EIF2AK3 and a review of the literature. Acta Paediatr 2004;93:1195–1201.
54 Delepine M, Nicolino M, Barrett T, Golamaully M, Lathrop GM, Julier C: EIF2AK3, encoding translation initiation factor 2-alpha kinase 3, is mutated in patients with Wolcott-Rallison syndrome. Nat Genet 2000;25:406–409.
55 Harding HP, Zhang Y, Bertolotti A, Zeng H, Ron D: Perk is essential for translational regulation and cell survival during the unfolded protein response. Mol Cell 2000;5:897–904.
56 Harding HP, Zeng H, Zhang Y, Jungries R, Chung P, Plesken H, et al: Diabetes mellitus and exocrine pancreatic dysfunction in perk–/– mice reveals a role for translational control in secretory cell survival. Mol Cell 2001;7:1153–1163.
57 Haines L, Wan KC, Lynn R, Barrett TG, Shield JP: Rising incidence of type 2 diabetes in children in the UK. Diabetes Care 2007;30:1097–1101.

Dr. Julian P. Hamilton-Shield
University of Bristol and Bristol Royal Hospital for Children, Upper Maudlin St.
Bristol BS2 8AE (UK)
Tel. +44 117 342 0159, Fax +44 117 342 0178, E-Mail j.p.h.shield@bristol.ac.uk

Shield JPH, Scharfmann R (eds): Development of the Pancreas and Neonatal Diabetes.
Endocr Dev. Basel, Karger, 2007, vol 12, pp 24–32

Transcription Factors in Pancreatic Development

Animal Models

Merce Martin • Viviane Hauer • Mélanie Messmer • Christophe Orvain • Gérard Gradwohl

Inserm U682, Development and Physiopathology of the Intestine and Pancreas, Université Louis Pasteur, Strasbourg, France

Abstract

Through the analysis of genetically modified mice a hierarchy of transcription factors regulating pancreas specification, endocrine destiny as well as endocrine subtype specification and differentiation has been established. In addition to conventional approaches such as transgenic technologies and gene targeting, recombinase fate mapping in mice has been key in establishing the lineage relationship between progenitor cells and their progeny in understanding pancreas formation. Moreover, the design of specific mouse models to conditionally express transcription factors in different populations of progenitor cells has revealed to what extent transcription factors required for islet cell development are also sufficient to induce endocrine differentiation and the importance of the competence of progenitor cells to respond to the genetic program implemented by these factors. Taking advantage of this basic science knowledge acquired in rodents, immature insulin-producing cells have recently been differentiated in vitro from human embryonic stem cells. Taken together these major advances emphasize the need to gain further in-depth knowledge of the molecular and cellular mechanisms controlling β-cell differentiation in mice to generate functional β-cells in the future that could be used for cell therapy in diabetes.

The adult pancreas consists of 3 principal tissue cell types all of endodermal origin: the exocrine acinar cells, the endocrine cells organized in islets (islets of Langerhans) and the ductal cells lining pancreatic ducts. In rodents, the first signs of pancreas organogenesis are the formation, at mid-gestation [embryonic day (E) 9–9.5], of two pancreatic buds (ventral and dorsal) in the region of the posterior foregut endoderm. The specification differentiation and growth of the two pancreatic buds are controlled by various signals originating from the adjacent mesodermal tissues. Dorsally, the pancreatic bud is sequentially exposed to signals from the notochord, dorsal aorta and pancreatic mesenchyme. Ventrally, both the cardiac mesoderm and vitellin veins control pancreas development. The two buds later fuse and the pancreatic epithelium branches and differentiates within the surrounding mesenchyme which further supports pancreatic growth. Concomitantly the different pancreatic cell types differentiate from immature pancreatic progenitor cells. During their differentiation endocrine precursors delaminate from the epithelium, migrate and aggregate in clusters called islets of Langerhans. Through the analysis of genetically modified mice, a complex hierarchy of transcription factors regulating pancreas organogenesis and islet cell differentiation has been established over the last few years. The purpose of this study is not to give an exhaustive list of these pancreatic transcription factors and their functions. For further information, excellent reviews have been published recently [1–3]. For the sake of simplicity, we will rather focus on describing how various important mouse models and sophisticated genetic tools, including loss and gain of function as well as lineage tracing approaches, have been in identifying the role of transcription factors in the control of key steps in pancreas and islet cell development.

Pancreas Specification and Growth

Two transcription factors, the genes *Pdx1* and *Ptf1a/p48*, regulate the very early steps of pancreas development. The homeobox gene *Pdx1/IPF1* is already expressed in the prepancreatic endoderm (E8.5–9) before any evidence of bud formation and persists in proliferating pancreatic epithelial cells at the bud stage (fig. 1a, b) and during subsequent branching of the epithelium [4, 5]. During β-cell development Pdx1 is later reexpressed in the mature β-cell where it controls the transcription of the insulin gene in the adult pancreas [6]. Knocking out Pdx1 results in pancreas agenesis [5]. Pancreatic buds form but then stop their development and regress suggesting that pancreas specification from the foregut endoderm is not altered but rather that Pdx1 controls early pancreas growth. Recently, powerful techniques have been developed in mice allowing us to determine the lineage relationship between populations of stem or progenitor cells and their descendants during organogenesis providing tools to understand how tissues are formed [7]. Briefly, the principle is to genetically and permanently tag a cell transiently expressing a transcription factor to follow its progeny. Using such a recombinase-based fate mapping approach, Gu et al. [8] demonstrated that adult exocrine and ductal cells derive from Pdx1-expressing pancreatic epithelial progenitor cells. Similarly all islet cells develop from Pdx1-positive progenitors. Interestingly, in the same study, using a sophistication of the lineage tracing approach where the labelling of Pdx1-positive cells can be induced temporally (at different developmental stages), the authors could also conclude that endocrine and acinar cells are generated from Pdx1-positive cells throughout embryogenesis. In contrast, Pdx1-positive progenitors giving rise to ducts develop around E10.

The basic helix-loop-helix transcription factor Ptf1a was initially thought to be required exclusively for exocrine cell differentiation, since this protein regulates the

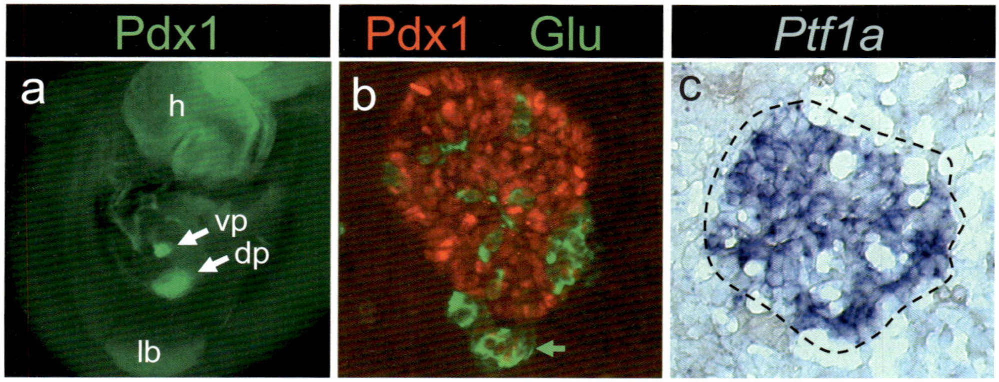

Fig. 1. Pdx1 and Ptf1a transcription factors control early steps of pancreas specification. **a** Whole-mount immunofluorescence for Pdx1 in an E10.5 mouse embryo revealing the formation of the ventral (vp) and dorsal pancreatic (dp) buds. h = Heart; lb = limb bud. **b** Immunofluorescence for Pdx1 and glucagon on a sagittal section through an E10.5 dorsal pancreatic bud showing the broad expression of Pdx1 in pancreatic epithelial progenitor cells as well as the formation of the first glucagon-expressing cells. **c** In situ hybridization revealing the expression of Ptf1a transcripts in pancreatic epithelial progenitor cells on a sagittal section of an E10.5 dorsal pancreatic bud. Dashed line limits the area of the dorsal pancreatic bud.

transcription of exocrine-specific genes such as α-amylase and exocrine cells are lacking in *Ptf1a*-deficient mice [9]. In 2002, Kawaguchi et al. [10] revisited the phenotype of Ptf1a knockout mice. Indeed, Chris Wright's laboratory has generated a very elegant knock-in mouse model where the progeny of Ptf1a-positive cells can be followed even in *Ptf1a*-deficient mice [10]. The authors replaced the Ptf1a coding sequence by the Cre recombinase using homologous recombination in embryonic stem cells. The resulting $Ptf1a^{+/Cre}$ mouse was crossed with the *Rosa26R* Cre reporter line where the transcription of the β-galactosidase gene is activated upon Cre-mediated excision of an upstream STOP cassette flanked by loxP sites. Consequently, Ptf1a-expressing cells and their progeny permanently express the β-galactosidase gene and can thus be identified. This experiment revealed that Ptf1a is, like Pdx1, largely expressed at the early bud stage in uncommitted pancreatic progenitors (fig. 1c). Accordingly, fate mapping of these Ptf1a-expressing cells demonstrated that Ptf1a-positive cells give rise to endocrine, ductal and acinar cells. In *Ptf1a*-deficient mice, the ventral pancreas was completely lacking and only a dorsal pancreatic rudiment could be found. Very interestingly, $Ptf1a^{Cre/Cre}$;*Rosa26R* mice revealed that in the absence of Ptf1a, the prospective ventral bud adopts an intestinal fate, demonstrating that Ptf1a is essential for pancreas specification in uncommitted foregut endodermal progenitor cells. Finally, recent data suggest that Ptf1a could be an activator of early Pdx1 expression in pancreas progenitors [11]. Taken together, Ptf1a and Pdx1 control specification and growth of the pancreatic buds. The downstream targets of these two transcription factors and potential effectors of their function remain largely to be identified.

Endocrine Cell Fate Commitment

When pancreatic progenitor cells have been specified and express the transcription factors Pdx1 and Ptf1a, their next important cell fate decision is whether they adopt an exocrine, ductal or endocrine destiny. We have recently demonstrated that the basic helix-loop-helix transcription factor Neurogenin 3 (Ngn3) is key in such decisions promoting an islet fate in Pdx1-positive pancreatic progenitor cells [12]. Indeed we initially showed that Ngn3 is expressed, from the bud stage, in immature cells in the developing pancreas that do not express either islet hormones or exocrine markers (fig. 2a). The number of Ngn3 cells peaks during the secondary transition phase and major wave of islet cell neogenesis (fig. 2b–d). Moreover, when Ngn3 was inactivated, mice died on postnatal days 1–3 and were severely diabetic lacking all islet cells (fig. 2e, f), demonstrating that Ngn3 is essential for islet cell development [12]. Provided that both in vertebrates and invertebrates transcription factors of the basic helix-loop-helix family regulate cell fate and differentiation in a cell-autonomous fashion, our data strongly suggest that the expression of Ngn3 in developing pancreatic cells determines their endocrine destiny. In other words, Ngn3 acts as a genetic switch inducing an endocrine fate in uncommitted pancreatic progenitor cells. Lineage tracing in mice later formally proved that α-glucagon-, β-insulin-, δ-somatostatin-, pancreatic polypeptide-, as well as the recently discovered ε-ghrelin-secreting cells arise from *Ngn3*-positive cells [8, 13]. Importantly, Ngn3 is not only essential for islet cell fate commitment but is also sufficient to promote pancreatic endocrine differentiation as α-, β-, δ-, and pancreatic polypeptide islet cells could be rescued by conditional and transient expression of Ngn3 in uncommitted Pdx1-expressing cells in a *Ngn3*-deficient background [14]. These experiments also revealed that pancreatic progenitor cells go through competence windows during embryogenesis for the Ngn3-induced generation of different islet cell types and that changes in competence are intrinsic to the epithelium and do not depend on extrinsic cues [14].

It is thus clear that the expression of Ngn3 in Pdx1-positive pancreatic progenitor cells is necessary and sufficient to determine their endocrine destiny. However, there are still some remaining and important questions like the differentiation potency of Ngn3-positive islet progenitor cells. Are these endocrine progenitors mono- or pluripotent? In other words, can a single Ngn3 cell give rise to one or several endocrine cell types? What are the signals inducing Ngn3 expression and the commitment of Ngn3-positive cells to one or the other islet cell lineages? Also the full set of Ngn3 target genes induced in vivo, in the developing pancreas is not known. To further understand the molecular and biological characteristics of islet progenitor cells we have generated mice where this cell population can be purified or followed in real time in embryonic pancreas explant cultures [15]. To find additional regulators of islet subtype specification and endocrine differentiation we have performed a series of DNA microarray hybridization experiments and determined the com-

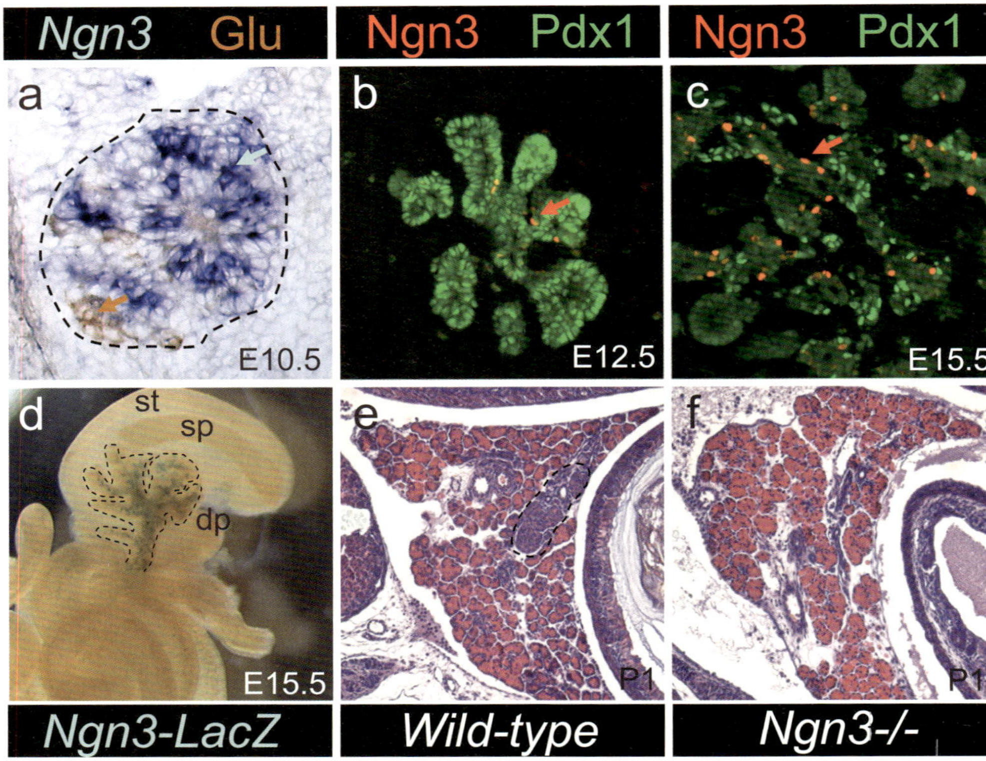

Fig. 2. Ngn3 controls endocrine destiny in pancreatic progenitor cells. **a** In situ hybridization showing Ngn3 transcript expression in immature endocrine cells (islet progenitor cells) that do not yet express hormones revealed by immunofluorescence for glucagon. **b**, **c** Double immunofluorescence for Pdx1 and Ngn3. Ngn3-positive islet progenitor cells (red arrows) arise from uncommitted Pdx1-positive epithelial cells and their number increases until E15.5. **d** β-Galactosidase activity in the digestive tract of an E15.5 Ngn3 (promoter)-LacZ transgenic mouse reveals islet progenitor cells (blue) in the branching dorsal pancreas (dp). st = Stomach; sp = spleen. **e**, **f** Hematoxylin-eosin staining on pancreas sections of P1 wild-type and Ngn3$^{-/-}$ mice. Islets of Langerhans do not form in the pancreas of Ngn3-deficient mice. Dashed line in **a** and **e** limits the area of the dorsal pancreatic bud and islet of Langerhans, respectively.

plete transcriptome of the purified islet progenitor cells as well as identified the panel of Ngn3 target genes [unpubl. data]. These studies have already led to the identification of the zinc finger transcription factor IA1/Insm1, a direct target of Ngn3, essential for the maturation of islet cells [16]. Additional known and unknown genes enriched in islet progenitor cells that are induced by Ngn3 and lost in Ngn3-deficient mice are currently being characterized. The identification of the function of these genes will be particularly relevant to decipher the Ngn3-dependent genetic programs controlling generic and subtype-specific properties of islet progenitor cells.

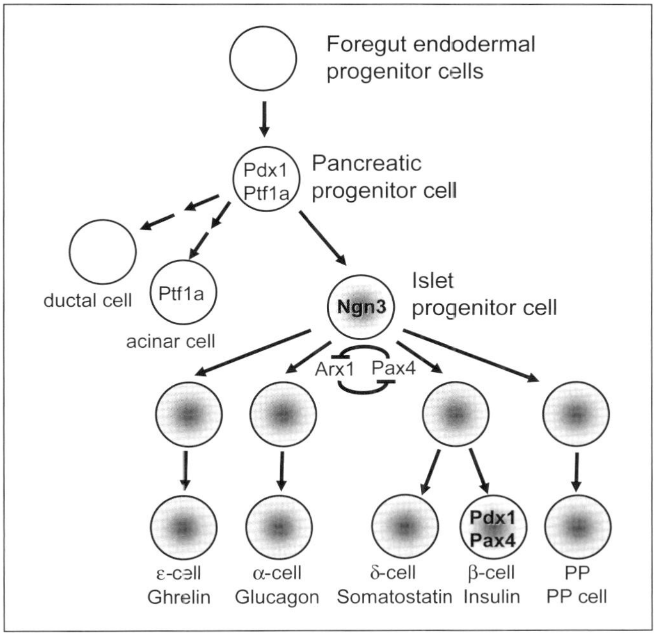

Fig. 3. Hierarchy of transcription factors controlling key steps in islet cell development. Simplified scheme based on spatiotemporal expression and phenotypic results of mouse models of loss- and gain-of-function studies and lineage tracing. PP = Pancreatic polypeptide.

Specification of the Different Islet Endocrine Cell Types

Although the complete endocrinogenic program implemented downstream of Ngn3 is not known, very significant progress has been obtained in the identification of transcription factor networks operating in developing islet cells regulating the progressive specification and maturation of endocrine subtype lineages as well as maintaining the differentiated phenotype. In this area, gene inactivation in mice, as well as gain-of-function studies have revealed the key and antagonistic functions of two homeodomain-containing proteins, the transcription factors Pax4 and aristaless-related homeobox (Arx), for proper islet cell specification. Briefly, *Arx*-deficient mice are hypoglycemic and die on day 2, α-cells are lost and the number of β- and δ-cells increases [17]. In contrast, *Pax4*-deficient mice are hyperglycemic, die on day 2, β- and δ-cells are lost and the number of α-cells increases [18]. Interestingly, *Arx* and *Pax4* transcript levels are increased in the embryonic pancreas of *Pax4*- and *Arx*-deficient mice, respectively [17]. Taken together, these findings suggest that during development, islet progenitor cells can either become precursors of β/δ-cells or α-cells and that these alternative fates are promoted by Pax4 and Arx, respectively (fig. 3). Moreover, these two transcription factors repress each other by direct interaction with their respective promoter region to control appropriate endocrine cell allocation. Interestingly, in *Pax4/Arx* double mutants, whereas both α- and β-cells are lost, somatostatin-expressing δ-cells develop normally, suggesting that Pax4 is not necessary for δ-cell genesis and induces a β-cell fate [19]. In a recent and very elegant series of Arx conditional misexpression experiments, Collombat et al. [20] further demonstrated that Arx is not only necessary but also sufficient to promote an α-cell fate in the embryonic pancreas. Even more spectacularly, misexpression of Arx in adult β-cells results in the loss of the β-cell phenotype and concomitant increase in the number of α-cells.

Taken together, these examples demonstrate that mouse models allowing inactivation or forced expression of specific genes or allowing us to follow the destiny of progenitor cells were instrumental in deciphering the complex mechanisms controlling the progressive restriction of endodermal stem/progenitor cells to highly differentiated islet cells with specialized functions.

From Developmental Biology towards a Cell Therapy for Diabetes

Understanding the mechanisms controlling multipotent stem cell differentiation into specialized cells during the embryonic life is not only one of the current challenges in stem cell biology but will also have a crucial impact on future cell replacement therapies designed to treat diseases such as type 1 diabetes. Currently available, exogenous insulin therapy for type 1 diabetes is not a panacea as it often fails to prevent the development of long-term comorbidities. Recently, transplantation of pancreatic islets, derived from allogeneic donors, achieved, to some extent, remission in insulin requirement in type 1 diabetes patients [21], providing a proof of concept for a cell-based therapy in diabetes. Of central importance for the development of such a therapy is the generation of sufficient and functional β-cells to circumvent the shortage of transplantable islets. Recent data support the concept that in the healthy adult mouse, the β-cell pool is maintained by replication of differentiated β-cells [22, 23]. However, the conditions for the in vitro expansion of functional β-cells are unknown. In contrast, during embryogenesis, de novo generated β-cells arise from pancreatic stem/progenitor cells. Therefore, understanding the molecular mechanisms underlying embryonic β-cell development is essential if we want to recapitulate a β-cell differentiation program and generate functional insulin-secreting cells for therapy starting from 'plastic' cells such as embryonic or somatic stem cells. Following this strategy, a Biotech company in California has recently been able to convert human embryonic stem cells into insulin-producing cells using a stepwise protocol based on pancreatic development [24]. Briefly, human embryonic stem cells were treated with soluble factors to mimic in vivo pancreas organogenesis by inducing successively: definitive endoderm, gut endoderm, pancreatic endoderm and endocrine precursors. Successful induction of these developmental stages was monitored by the expression of specific transcription factors including those described above. Despite this important progress, the insulin-producing cells generated are still immature and remain different from normal glucose-responsive single-hormone-positive human islet β-cells [25]. These seminal studies from Baetge's laboratory provide a proof of principle for the generation of β-cells from human embryonic stem cells and underline the biomedical relevance of mouse models to decipher the functions of transcription factors in islet cell development. However, this study also highlights the critical importance of continuing such basic research to gain a deeper knowledge of the network of transcription factors and their targets controlling not only islet cell fate decisions but also islet cell maturation and islet morphogenesis. In the future, this knowledge will in turn be instrumental in successfully generating in vitro, not only β-cells but also therapeutic islets that very likely would confer a better regulation of glucose homeostasis in transplanted patients.

Acknowledgments

Research projects performed in the laboratory received financial support from Inserm, the French National Research Program for Diabetes (PNRD), the Juvenile Diabetes Research Foundation (JDRF), the EU (Integrated project 6th FP 'Betacelltherapy' to the JDRF Center) and the NIH Beta Cell Biology Consortium (DK072495-01).

References

1 Habener JF, Kemp DM, Thomas MK: Minireview: Transcriptional regulation in pancreatic development. Endocrinology 2005;146:1025–1034.

2 Collombat P, Hecksher-Sorensen J, Serup P, Mansouri A: Specifying pancreatic endocrine cell fates. Mech Dev 2006;123:501–512.

3 Murtaugh LC: Pancreas and beta-cell development: from the actual to the possible. Development 2007;134:427–438.

4 Ahlgren U, Jonsson J, Edlund H: The morphogenesis of the pancreatic mesenchyme is uncoupled from that of the pancreatic epithelium in IPF1/PDX1-deficient mice. Development 1996;122:1409–1416.

5 Offield MF, Jetton TL, Labosky PA, Ray M, Stein RW, Magnuson MA, Hogan BL, Wright CV: PDX-1 is required for pancreatic outgrowth and differentiation of the rostral duodenum. Development 1996;122:983–995.

6 Ohlsson H, Karlsson K, Edlund T: IPF1, a homeodomain-containing transactivator of the insulin gene. EMBO J 1993;12:4251–4259.

7 Furuta Y, Behringer RR: Recent innovations in tissue-specific gene modifications in the mouse. Birth Defects Res C Embryo Today 2005;75:43–57.

8 Gu G, Dubauskaite J, Melton DA: Direct evidence for the pancreatic lineage: NGN3+ cells are islet progenitors and are distinct from duct progenitors. Development 2002;129:2447–2457.

9 Krapp A, Knofler M, Ledermann B, Burki K, Berney C, Zoerkler N, Hagenbuchle O, Wellauer PK: The bHLH protein PTF1-p48 is essential for the formation of the exocrine and the correct spatial organization of the endocrine pancreas. Genes Dev 1998;12:3752–3763.

10 Kawaguchi Y, Cooper B, Gannon M, Ray M, MacDonald RJ, Wright CV: The role of the transcriptional regulator Ptf1a in converting intestinal to pancreatic progenitors. Nat Genet 2002;32:128–134.

11 Wiebe PO, Kormish JD, Roper VT, Fujitani Y, Alston NI, Zaret KS, Wright CV, Stein RW, Gannon M: Ptf1a binds to and activates area III, a highly conserved region of the Pdx1 promoter that mediates early pancreas-wide Pdx1 expression. Mol Cell Biol 2007;27:4093–4104.

12 Gradwohl G, Dierich A, LeMeur M, Guillemot F: Neurogenin3 is required for the development of the four endocrine cell lineages of the pancreas. Proc Natl Acad Sci USA 2000;97:1607–1611.

13 Heller RS, Jenny M, Collombat P, Mansouri A, Tomasetto C, Madsen OD, Mellitzer G, Gradwohl G, Serup P: Genetic determinants of pancreatic epsilon-cell development. Dev Biol 2005;286:217–224.
14 Johansson KA, Dursun U, Jordan N, Gu G, Beermann F, Gradwohl G, Grapin-Botton A: Temporal control of neurogenin3 activity in pancreas progenitors reveals competence windows for the generation of different endocrine cell types. Dev Cell 2007;12:457–465.
15 Mellitzer G, Martin M, Sidhoum-Jenny M, Orvain C, Barths J, Seymour PA, Sander M, Gradwohl G: Pancreatic islet progenitor cells in neurogenin 3-yellow fluorescent protein knock-add-on mice. Mol Endocrinol 2004;18:2765–2776.
16 Mellitzer G, Bonne S, Luco RF, Van De CM, Lenne-Samuel N, Collombat P, Mansouri A, Lee J, Lan M, Pipeleers D, Nielsen FC, Ferrer J, Gradwohl G, Heimberg H: IA1 is NGN3-dependent and essential for differentiation of the endocrine pancreas. EMBO J 2006;25:1344–1352.
17 Collombat P, Mansouri A, Hecksher-Sorensen J, Serup P, Krull J, Gradwohl G, Gruss P: Opposing actions of Arx and Pax4 in endocrine pancreas development. Genes Dev 2003;17:2591–2603.
18 Sosa-Pineda B, Chowdhury K, Torres M, Oliver G, Gruss P: The Pax4 gene is essential for differentiation of insulin-producing beta cells in the mammalian pancreas. Nature 1997;386:399–402.
19 Collombat P, Hecksher-Sorensen J, Broccoli V, Krull J, Ponte I, Mundiger T, Smith J, Gruss P, Serup P, Mansouri A: The simultaneous loss of Arx and Pax4 genes promotes a somatostatin-producing cell fate specification at the expense of the alpha- and beta-cell lineages in the mouse endocrine pancreas. Development 2005;132:2969–2980.
20 Collombat P, Hecksher-Sorensen J, Krull J, Berger J, Riedel D, Herrera PL, Serup P, Mansouri A: Embryonic endocrine pancreas and mature beta cells acquire alpha and PP cell phenotypes upon Arx misexpression. J Clin Invest 2007;117:961–970.
21 Shapiro AM, Lakey JR, Ryan EA, Korbutt GS, Toth E, Warnock GL, Kneteman NM, Rajotte RV: Islet transplantation in seven patients with type 1 diabetes mellitus using a glucocorticoid-free immunosuppressive regimen. N Engl J Med 2000;343:230–238.
22 Dor Y, Brown J, Martinez OI, Melton DA: Adult pancreatic beta-cells are formed by self-duplication rather than stem-cell differentiation. Nature 2004;429:41–46.
23 Brennand K, Huangfu D, Melton D: All beta cells contribute equally to islet growth and maintenance. PLoS Biol 2007;5:e163.
24 D'Amour KA, Bang AG, Eliazer S, Kelly OG, Agulnick AD, Smart NG, Moorman MA, Kroon E, Carpenter MK, Baetge EE: Production of pancreatic hormone-expressing endocrine cells from human embryonic stem cells. Nat Biotechnol 2006;24:1392–1401.
25 Madsen OD, Serup P: Towards cell therapy for diabetes. Nat Biotechnol 2006;24:1481–1483.

Dr. Gérard Gradwohl
INSERM U682, Development and Physiopathology of the Intestine and Pancreas, Université Louis Pasteur
3, avenue Molière, FR–67200 Strasbourg (France)
Tel. +33 3 88 27 5366, Fax +33 3 88 26 3538, E-Mail gerard.gradwohl@inserm.u-strasbg.fr

Shield JPH, Scharfmann R (eds): Development of the Pancreas and Neonatal Diabetes.
Endocr Dev. Basel, Karger, 2007, vol 12, pp 33–45

Distinct Roles of HNF1β, HNF1α, and HNF4α in Regulating Pancreas Development, β-Cell Function and Growth

Miguel Angel Maestro · Carina Cardalda · Sylvia F. Boj · Reini F. Luco · Joan Marc Servitja · Jorge Ferrer

Genomic Programming of Beta Cells Laboratory, Institut d'Investigacions Biomèdiques August Pi i Sunyer, Endocrinology, Hospital Clínic de Barcelona, Barcelona, Spain

Abstract

Mutations in the genes encoding transcriptional regulators HNF1β (TCF2), HNF1α (TCF1), and HNF4α cause autosomal dominant diabetes (also known as maturity-onset diabetes of the young). Herein, we review what we have learnt during recent years concerning the functions of these regulators in the developing and adult pancreas. Mouse studies have revealed that HNF1β is a critical regulator of a transcriptional network that controls the specification, growth, and differentiation of the embryonic pancreas. HNF1β mutations in humans accordingly often cause pancreas hypoplasia. By contrast, HNF1α and HNF4α have been shown to regulate the function of differentiated β-cells. HNF1α and HNF4α mutations in patients thus cause decreased glucose-induced insulin secretion that leads to a progressive form of diabetes. HNF4α mutations paradoxically also cause in utero and neonatal hyperinsulinism, which later evolves to decreased glucose-induced secretion. Recent studies show that *Hnf4a* deficiency in mice causes not only abnormal insulin secretion, but also an impairment of the expansion of β-cell mass that normally occurs during pregnancy. In line with this finding, we present data that *Hnf1a*$^{-/-}$ β-cells expressing SV40 large T antigen show a severe impairment of proliferation and failure to form tumours. Collectively, these findings implicate HNF1β as a regulator of pancreas organogenesis and differentiation, whereas HNF1α and HNF4α primarily regulate both growth and function of islet β-cells.

More than 70 years ago, a form of diabetes was described that develops in young individuals and is inherited in an autosomal dominant manner [1]. Several decades later, Fajans and Conn [2] and Tattersall [3] coined the term 'maturity-onset diabetes of the young' (MODY), and introduced criteria that are currently still employed to define this entity clinically, namely: (a) a diagnosis before 25 years of age in at least one family member; (b) autosomal dominant inheritance pattern with high pheno-

Table 1. Genetic classification of autosomal dominant diabetes (MODY)

Locus	Gene name	Gene symbols	Gene class	Clinical phenotype
MODY1	Hepatic nuclear factor 4α	*HNF4A*[1], HNF4α	Transcription factor (nuclear receptor)	Diabetes; neonatal hyperinsulinism
MODY2	Glucokinase	*GCK*	Hexokinase	Mild hyperglycaemia
MODY3	Hepatic nuclear factor 1α	HNF1α, *TCF1*	Transcription factor (homeodomain)	Diabetes
MODY4	Insulin promoter factor 1	*IPF1,* PDX1, SFT1, IDX1	Transcription factor (homeodomain)	Diabetes; pancreas agenesis in homozygosity
MODY5	Hepatic nuclear factor 1β	HNF1β, vHNF1, *TCF2*	Transcription factor (homeodomain)	Diabetes; pancreas hypoplasia; renal/genitourinary malformations
MODY6	NEUROD1	*NEUROD1,* BETA2	Transcription factor (bHLH)	Diabetes

[1] The official human gene symbol is italicized.

typic penetrance, and (c) lack of evidence of severe insulin deficiency during initial phases of the disease [2, 3]. During the 1990s, several genes involved in MODY were identified, primarily through the use of positional cloning strategies [4–12]. This revealed that MODY is in fact a heterogeneous entity from both clinical and molecular genetic standpoints (table 1). In one group of patients, mutations in the glycolytic enzyme glucokinase were found to cause familial mild hyperglycaemia [5, 6, 13]. A different phenotype with full-blown diabetes was found to result from mutations in *HNF1α (TCF1)* or *HNF4α* genes [10–12, 14, 15]. A third group of patients carried mutations in *HNF1β (TCF2),* and had a syndromic form of diabetes that is associated with other developmental abnormalities [7, 16, 17]. Finally, other rare but biologically insightful forms of diabetes are caused by mutations in transcription factors IPF1 and NEUROD1 [8, 9].

HNF1β, HNF4α, and *HNF1α* are clearly the most prevalent culprits of transcription factor autosomal dominant diabetes. These 3 genes also share the fact that their role in regulating glucose homeostasis was unsuspected prior to the discovery of the genetic causes of MODY. In this chapter, we focus on recent advances in our understanding of the biological functions of HNF1β, HNF4α, and HNF1α in pancreatic β-cells. We relate these findings to the pathophysiology of MODY and discuss clinical implications, but refer readers to other reviews for a comprehensive overview of the molecular genetics and clinical presentation of MODY [18].

The Maturity-Onset Diabetes of the Young Type 5 Gene Product HNF1β (TCF2) Regulates Pancreas Specification, Morphogenesis, and Differentiation

Although first identified as a monogenic diabetes gene, heterozygous *HNF1β* mutations also cause renal cystic disease, cholestatic jaundice, and diverse genitourinary abnormalities [7, 16, 17, 19–21]. There is considerable heterogeneity in the phenotype, even within families, and thus no obvious relationship to the nature of the mutation.

The search for mutations in HNF1β in MODY was based on its structural resemblance to the MODY3 gene product HNF1α [7]. It was thus based on intelligent intuition, rather than on any preconceived knowledge of the biological functions of HNF1β in relation to the regulation of glucose homeostasis or β-cell development. It was only some years after the discovery of MODY5 that it became clear that HNF1β is not even expressed at significant levels in β-cells, but is specifically enriched in the early pancreatic endoderm [22]. As pancreas development progresses, HNF1β protein expression is restricted to highly proliferative epithelial cells that line both large and small ducts [22]. Immunofluorescence colabelling studies showed that endocrine-committed progenitors expressing Ngn3 appear to originate from this HNF1β-expressing epithelium, strongly suggesting that HNF1β marks a pool of precursor cells that gives rise to endocrine cells, and most likely also acinar and adult duct cells. HNF1β in fact turned out to be the first transcription factor shown to be selectively expressed within the embryonic pancreas.

Genetic studies to assess the possible functional role of HNF1β in the developing pancreas were initially hampered by the fact that $Hnf1\beta^{+/-}$ mice exhibit no apparent phenotype, while homozygous Hnf1β mutations result in embryonic lethality prior to the formation of the pancreas [23, 24]. The latter is due to defective gastrulation resulting from the essential role of HNF1β in extra-embryonic membranes [23, 24]. In an elegant approach to circumvent this difficulty, the Cereghini laboratory generated chimeric mice where the extra-embryonic membranes expressed Hnf1β, while embryonic cells were $Hnf1\beta^{-/-}$ [25]. Hnf1β-deficient embryos were shown to have no detectable ventral pancreas, and failed to express several key early pancreatic endoderm markers such as Pdx1, Ptf1, and Hlxb9 at the site where the ventral pancreas is formed [25]. A very small dorsal pancreas was nonetheless formed. These dorsal bud cells failed to proliferate, and did not form the characteristic ductal branching pattern. Moreover, the dorsal pancreas in Hnf1β-deficient embryos failed to express Ngn3 and did not form endocrine cells [25]. HNF1β has also been shown to regulate HNF6 (Onecut1), an indispensable factor for the proper differentiation of Ngn3-expressing cells, while Hnf6-deficient embryos in turn exhibit a severe reduction of HNF1β expression in pancreatic ducts and biliary cells [22, 26, 27]. Taken together, these findings show that HNF1β is a marker of early and late pancreatic precursor cells, and more importantly that it is an essential regulator of the transcriptional networks that control the specification of the pancreas, its morphogenesis, and the differentiation of endocrine cells.

Parallel studies in humans with MODY5 have shown a comparable role of HNF1β in pancreas organogenesis. Computerized tomography studies revealed pancreatic hypoplasia in 5/6 subjects with MODY5, and patients with this disease can present not only diabetes but also mild exocrine dysfunction [16]. Similarly pancreas hypoplasia with complete absence of ventral-derived tissue and perturbed morphogenesis was encountered in fetuses with HNF1β mutations [28]. In keeping with this notion, while MODY5 is detected after the first decade in most patients, rare patients with more severe pancreatic expressivity of HNF1β mutations present with neonatal diabetes and exocrine dysfunction [21, 29].

The Maturity-Onset Diabetes of the Young Type 3 Gene Product HNF1α (TCF1) Regulates Differentiated β-Cell Functions

Patients with HNF1α mutations develop diabetes after the first decade, and it is preceded by abnormal glucose-induced insulin secretion [30, 31]. The penetrance is high, although it is dependent on age, so that the probability of being diagnosed with diabetes increases steadily between 10 and 50 years of age [14, 18]. It is not clear why different individuals develop diabetes at diverse ages, or why the severity of β-cell dysfunction differs substantially. So far, no conclusive evidence has been reported that obesity or sedentary lifestyle is a decisive factor. Disease severity varies according to the location of mutations, such that mutations in exons 8–10 of HNF1α, which interestingly turn out to form part of a splice variant that is comparatively less abundant in islets, have a later diagnosis [32].

Unlike what is observed for HNF1β mutations, there are no clinically apparent associated developmental abnormalities in MODY3, and no signs of pancreatic hypoplasia have been reported. MODY3 patients have nonetheless been found to have subtle associated defects such as a decreased threshold for glycosuria reflecting renal tubular dysfunction [33].

The HNF1α-deficient phenotype in MODY3 patients is consistent with other knowledge indicating that HNF1α predominantly regulates differentiated cellular functions, rather than developmental processes. HNF1α is a homeodomain protein that is structurally very closely related to HNF1β. Both proteins share very similar DNA binding and dimerization domains, allowing them to form either homo- or heterodimers. One explanation for the divergent functions despite the structural similarities is that their cellular expression domains are quite distinct [34]. For example, whilst HNF1β is expressed in pancreatic embryonic precursor cells and adult ducts, HNF1α is enriched in acinar and endocrine differentiated cells [22, 35].

Unlike in humans, heterozygous HNF1α mutations in mice do not give rise to an obvious phenotype. Homozygous mutations, although not strictly a model for human disease, provide a very powerful tool to understand the function of HNF1α. *Hnf1α*$^{-/-}$

mice have no gross developmental defects, but have severe dysfunction of hepatocytes, renal tubular cells, and β-cells, and thus develop diabetes [36–38]. Detailed studies of β-cell function in *Hnf1α*$^{-/-}$ mice have revealed a severe abrogation of glucose-induced insulin secretion [38, 39]. This is in part linked to defective islet-cell glycolytic flux, and is associated with decreased expression of Glut2 glucose transporter and L-type pyruvate kinase genes in both *Hnf1α*$^{-/-}$ mice and in INS1 cells expressing a dominant negative inhibitor of HNF1α [40–42]. Another gene potentially involved in the HNF1α-deficient secretory defect is collectrin/Tmem27, a gene that has been implicated in the regulation of either exocytosis or β-cell growth [43, 44]. A different source of information on HNF1α targets comes from chromatin immunoprecipitation analysis of microarrays containing more than 10,000 promoter regions [45]. This impressive study revealed that HNF1α binds to a large number of genes that encode for a broad spectrum of functional categories, including many involved in diverse metabolic functions [45]. Although most such genes that are bound by HNF1α are not necessarily functionally dependent on HNF1α, large-scale gene expression studies in *Hnf1α*$^{-/-}$ islets demonstrate that HNF1α indeed regulates diverse islet cell functions, rather than a discrete signalling pathway [J.M.S., unpubl. results]. Both chromatin immunoprecipitation and expression studies also coincide in showing that HNF1α regulates a network of pancreatic islet transcription factors, including HNF4γ and the MODY1 gene *HNF4α* [45, 46].

Pearson and Hattersley have exploited knowledge of HNF1α function in β-cells to provide a fascinating example of translational pharmacogenomics [47–49]. Noting that early steps in stimulus-secretion coupling in *Hnf1α*$^{-/-}$ islets are defective, while insulin gene expression and K_{ATP} channel expression are not grossly altered, a randomized therapeutic trial with sulphonylureas was carried out in MODY3 patients [48]. This revealed that MODY3 patients are uniquely sensitive to sulphonylureas, much more so than patients with polygenic type 2 diabetes [48]. This observation has modified therapeutic recommendations in MODY3, enabling successful diabetes treatment with sulphonylureas in many MODY3 patients, often in patients who had previously been on insulin therapy for decades [47].

Regulation of β-Cell Growth by HNF1α

Although defects in β-cell stimulus-secretion coupling in *Hnf1α*-deficient MODY are unquestionable, the progressive nature of MODY3 is also consistent with a simultaneous defect in the ability to increase β-cell mass to match increasing demands. Studies in *Hnf1α*-deficient mice, however, have not provided conclusive results in this regard. No reduction in β-cell mass in *Hnf1α*$^{+/-}$ mice has been reported, and although β-cell mass is reduced in *Hnf1α*$^{-/-}$ islets, it is not inappropriately decreased when the severely diminished weight of these mice is taken into consideration [38]. Furthermore, although expression of dominant negative HNF1α in β-cells results in a severe reduction of β-cell mass, overexpression of the wild-type version of HNF1α unexpectedly also results in a comparably severe phenotype [50, 51].

We have measured the proportion of β-cells relative to other pancreatic cells in very young (2-week-old) mice to circumvent possible confounding consequences of prolonged diabetes and metabolic abnormalities, and noted no major differences relative to wild-type mice (fig. 1a). However, a clear reduction in the size of pancreatic islets was noted that is compensated by a larger number of extra-insular β-cells or small clusters (fig. 1b, c). We also measured proliferation rates in embryonic day 18.5 embryos, where blood glucose is normal in all genotypes, and in 3-month-old mice (fig. 1d–f). Although lower than average values were noted in $Hnf1\alpha^{-/-}$ β-cells, this did not reach statistical significance (fig. 1d–f).

Studies to address the ability of $Hnf1\alpha^{-/-}$ mice to increase β-cell mass with ageing or in response to increased metabolic demands are nearly impossible to carry out and interpret, because these mice have a high mortality and suffer from liver and kidney dysfunction as well as diabetes [36, 37]. We have used one possible approach to study stimulated β-cell growth by generating mice expressing the SV40 T antigen oncogene selectively in pancreatic β-cells under the control of the rat insulin II promoter (Rip2-TAg) on either $Hnf1\alpha^{+/+}$, $Hnf1\alpha^{+/-}$, or $Hnf1\alpha^{-/-}$ backgrounds. As expected [52, 53], the Rip2-TAg transgene invariably caused insulinomas after 3 months of age on both $Hnf1\alpha^{+/+}$ and $Hnf1\alpha^{+/-}$ backgrounds, and this led to hypoglycaemia and death (fig. 1d, e). However, on an $Hnf1\alpha^{-/-}$ background the development of tumours was exceptional, it was observed only after 9 months, and tumour size at this time was more than 2-fold smaller than in $Hnf1\alpha^{+/+}$ or $Hnf1\alpha^{+/-}$ littermates at 12 weeks (fig. 1d, e). Although several factors could theoretically account for such reduced tumourgenicity, it was found to be in part due to reduced proliferation. Thus, in situ analysis of pancreatic tissues revealed that Ki67 labelling was reduced by 3-fold in T-antigen-expressing β-cells from $Hnf1\alpha^{-/-}$ Rip2-TAg versus $Hnf1\alpha^{+/+}$ Rip2-TAg mice (fig. 1f). Furthermore, whereas explanted $Hnf1\alpha^{+/+}$ Rip2-TAg β-cell lines exhibited a robust expansion in culture, dissected $Hnf1\alpha^{-/-}$ Rip2-TAg tumour cells placed in culture showed a complete failure to grow (fig. 1g). These results thus show that HNF1α is essential for the proliferative response that is induced by the T antigen oncogene in β-cells, and more generally they indicate that HNF1α controls cellular processes required for oncogenesis in β-cells. While this model differs from the physiological context of MODY3 patients, it suggests that impaired β-cell growth may form part of the pathophysiology of this disease.

The Maturity-Onset Diabetes of the Young Type 1 Gene Product HNF4α Regulates β-Cell Function and Growth

Clinically the diabetic phenotype in MODY1 is virtually indistinguishable from that due to HNF1α mutations (MODY3) [10, 18, 54–57]. In both forms of MODY patients develop a progressive form of diabetes after the first decade, with similar age-depen-

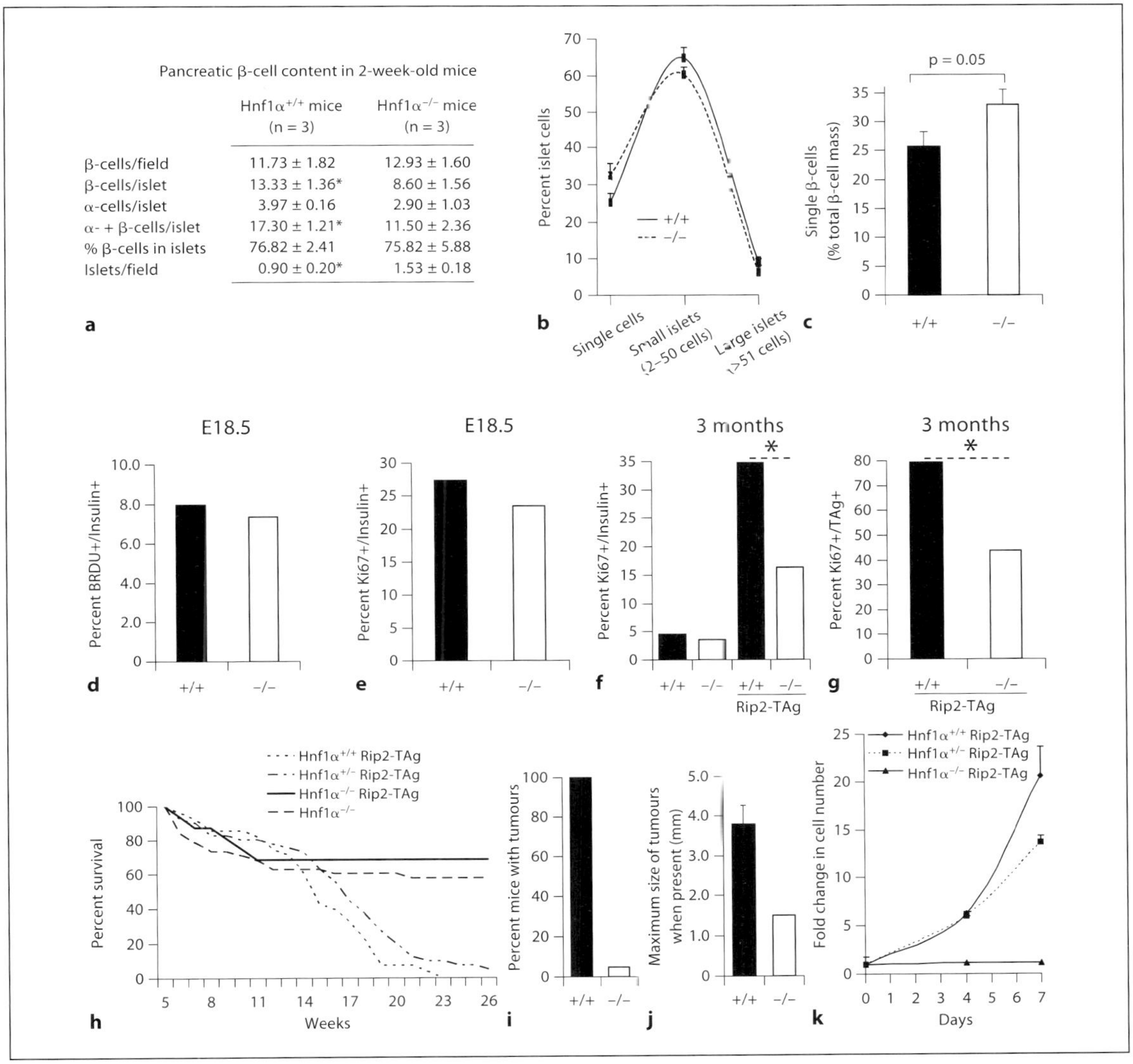

	Hnf1α$^{+/+}$ mice (n = 3)	Hnf1α$^{-/-}$ mice (n = 3)
β-cells/field	11.73 ± 1.82	12.93 ± 1.60
β-cells/islet	13.33 ± 1.36*	8.60 ± 1.56
α-cells/islet	3.97 ± 0.16	2.90 ± 1.03
α- + β-cells/islet	17.30 ± 1.21*	11.50 ± 2.36
% β-cells in islets	76.82 ± 2.41	75.82 ± 5.88
Islets/field	0.90 ± 0.20*	1.53 ± 0.18

Fig. 1. β-Cell growth in *Hnf1α*-deficient β-cells. **a** Summary of islet cell number counts in 3 non-consecutive sections from 3 2-week-old mice with indicated genotypes. **b, c** Percentage of β-cells among dispersed extra-insular β-cells, small islets, and large islets in both genotypes. **d, e** Percentage of β-cells that are BRDU+ or Ki67+ in embryonic day 18.5 embryos with indicated genotypes. **f** Percentage of β-cells that are Ki67+ in 3-month-old mice with indicated genotypes. **g** Percentage of T antigen+ (TAg+) cells that are Ki67+ in 3-month-old mice with indicated genotypes. **h** Survival curves of mice with indicated phenotypes, showing that the Rip2-TAg transgene does not lead to increased mortality when present on an *Hnf1α*$^{-/-}$ background. **i** Percentage of Rip-TAg mice with insulinomas. **j** The maximum tumour size, when one is found, on indicated *Hnf1α* genotype backgrounds. Note that for the *Hnf1α*$^{+/+}$ genetic background this analysis was carried out in 12-week-old mice, while in *Hnf1α*$^{-/-}$ mice, where no tumours were observed in 8 12-week-old mice, this analysis was carried out at 8–9 months of age. **k** In vitro growth curves of β-cell lines explanted from Rip2-TAg insulinomas from indicated *Hnf1α* locus genetic backgrounds. Cells were obtained as described in Efrat et al. [52], plated at 1×10^4 or 1×10^5 per well, and replicate wells were trypsinized at indicated days for cell counting. Note that the *Hnf1α*$^{-/-}$ Rip2-TAg cells derived from 2 tumours exhibit a complete failure to grow in culture. Asterisks indicate $p < 0.01$ using the χ^2 test.

dent penetrance curves, blunted glucose-induced insulin secretion, and a unique ability to respond to sulphonylurea drugs [10, 18, 54–57].

This shared phenotype is consistent with HNF1α and HNF4α forming part of a common regulatory network in β-cells [41, 45, 58–61]. It is now known that HNF1α is an essential regulator of HNF4α gene transcription in pancreatic cells, an effect that is mediated through the P2 pancreas-selective HNF4α promoter [46, 57, 59, 61]. Chromatin immunoprecipitation, cell culture, and genetic studies show that HNF4α in turn regulates the HNF1α promoter [45, 62–65], although specifically in islets the functional role of this interaction remains to be proven given that HNF1α expression in *Hnf4α*-deficient mouse islets is normal [66–68]. A further level of interdependence is strongly suggested by several observations that HNF4α and HNF1α can also establish protein-protein interactions [45, 69, 70].

The gene targets of HNF4α in β-cells that may account for the MODY1 phenotype remain to be fully explored. As with HNF1α, heterozygous *Hnf4α* mutations in mice do not lead to glucose intolerance or diabetes. Homozygous germ line *Hnf4α* mutations lead to very early embryonic lethality during gastrulation, before the pancreas is even formed [71]. To study HNF4α function in β-cells, different groups have used Cre/LoxP technology to inactivate the *Hnf4α* gene specifically in β-cells [66–68]. Mice with β-cell-specific ablation of the *Hnf4α* gene develop intraperitoneal glucose intolerance, and in two of three studies this was paradoxically associated with basal mildly reduced blood glucose and increased insulin levels [66–68]. One study suggested that this phenotype may be associated with decreased mRNA expression of the K_{ATP} channel subunit Kir6.2, although altered expression of Kir6.2 has not been confirmed in two other studies [66–68]. Importantly, the two studies that have examined islet function ex vivo showed diminished glucose-induced insulin secretion, confirming that HNF4α is an essential regulator of this function [66, 67].

Although entirely unexpected, the mildly increased basal insulin levels in β-cell *Hnf4α*-deficient mice have an interesting correlate in humans. Even though the MODY1 and MODY3 diabetic phenotypes are extremely similar, HNF4α mutation carriers present a distinct prediabetic phenotype that is clearly not observed in HNF1α carriers. Birth weight in HNF4α mutation carriers is on average 790 g higher than in siblings who do not carry the mutation, and there is frequently transient, neonatal hypoglycaemia [68]. This is paralleled by the observation that mice with β-cell-specific inactivation of *Hnf4α* exhibit increased insulin levels in utero and neonatally, and have markedly lower blood glucose levels at birth [68]. These unexpected results indicate that HNF4α deficiency paradoxically causes hyperinsulinism in utero and in the neonatal period, which later evolves to diabetes due to reduced insulin secretion. Because this is not observed in HNF1α carriers [68], it indicates that during these early stages HNF4α plays a role that is independent of HNF1α.

While β-cell mass under normal conditions is unaltered in β-cell-specific *Hnf4α* knockout mice, the Kaestner laboratory has shown that there is a defect in the increase in β-cell mass that normally occurs during pregnancy [72]. Microarray analysis suggested that downregulation of suppression of tumourigenicity 5 *(ST5)* mRNA may be a mediator of this effect [72]. On the other hand, our own studies have shown that wild-type and *Hnf4α*-deficient mice do not differ in the degree of deterioration of glucose tolerance occurring after 5-month treatment with a high-fat (54%) diet [S.F.B., unpubl. results]. Because high fat is a potent inductor of β-cell mass in mice, this suggests that defective β-cell growth in *Hnf4α*-deficient mice during pregnancy might be pathway-specific. Collectively, available data indicate that both HNF1α and HNF4α can regulate β-cell growth. Although this has been shown under very specific conditions, it suggests that abnormal β-cell growth may contribute to the diabetic phenotype that ensues with time in MODY1 and MODY3 mutation carriers.

Concluding Remarks

Human genetics has identified mutations in transcription factor genes that cause abnormal β-cell function and diabetes. This has led to a novel clinical and molecular classification of autosomal dominant diabetes, and enabled the study of the underlying pathophysiology. Major changes in therapeutic recommendations for many patients are one immediate result of these discoveries. In addition, this new knowledge has been decisive in uncovering unsuspected regulators of human β-cell development, function, and growth. Cellular and mouse genetic tools are now being used to understand the detailed mechanisms whereby monogenic diabetes genes control these processes, providing biological information that is potentially relevant for all forms of diabetes.

Acknowledgements

The authors' research is supported by the Juvenile Diabetes Research Foundation, the European Union Sixth Framework Programme, Instituto de Salud Carlos III, the European Foundation for the Study of Diabetes, and the Ministerio de Educación y Ciencia.

References

1 Cammidge PJ: Diabetes mellitus and heredity. Br Med J 1928;2:739.

2 Fajans SS, Conn JW: Tolbutamide-induced improvement in carbohydrate tolerance of young people with mild diabetes mellitus. Diabetes 1960;9: 83–88.

3 Tattersall RB: Mild familial diabetes with dominant inheritance. Q J Med 1974;43:339–357.

4 Bell GI, Xiang KS, Newman MV, Wu SH, Wright LG, Fajans SS, Spielman RS, Cox NJ: Gene for non-insulin-dependent diabetes mellitus (maturity-onset diabetes of the young subtype) is linked to DNA polymorphism on human chromosome 20q. Proc Natl Acad Sci USA 1991;88:1484–1488.

5 Froguel P, Vaxillaire M, Sun F, Velho G, Zouali H, Butel MO, Lesage S, Vionnet N, Clement K, Fougerousse F, et al: Close linkage of glucokinase locus on chromosome 7p to early-onset non-insulin-dependent diabetes mellitus. Nature 1992;356:162–164.

6 Hattersley AT, Turner RC, Permutt MA, Patel P, Tanizawa Y, Chiu KC, O'Rahilly S, Watkins PJ, Wainscoat JS: Linkage of type 2 diabetes to the glucokinase gene. Lancet 1992;339:1307–1310.
7 Horikawa Y, Iwasaki N, Hara M, Furuta H, Hinokio Y, Cockburn BN, Lindner T, Yamagata K, Ogata M, Tomonaga O, Kuroki H, Kasahara T, Iwamoto Y, Bell GI: Mutation in hepatocyte nuclear factor-1 beta gene (TCF2) associated with MODY. Nat Genet 1997;17:384–385.
8 Malecki MT, Jhala US, Antonellis A, Fields L, Doria A, Orban T, Saad M, Warram JH, Montminy M, Krolewski AS: Mutations in NEUROD1 are associated with the development of type 2 diabetes mellitus. Nat Genet 1999;23:323–328.
9 Stoffers DA, Ferrer J, Clarke WL, Habener JF: Early-onset type-II diabetes mellitus (MODY4) linked to IPF1. Nat Genet 1997;17:138–139.
10 Yamagata K, Furuta H, Oda N, Kaisaki PJ, Menzel S, Cox NJ, Fajans SS, Signorini S, Stoffel M, Bell GI: Mutations in the hepatocyte nuclear factor-4alpha gene in maturity-onset diabetes of the young (MODY1). Nature 1996;384:458–460.
11 Yamagata K, Oda N, Kaisaki PJ, Menzel S, Furuta H, Vaxillaire M, Southam L, Cox RD, Lathrop GM, Boriraj VV, Chen X, Cox NJ, Oda Y, Yano H, Le Beau MM, Yamada S, Nishigori H, Takeda J, Fajans SS, Hattersley AT, Iwasaki N, Hansen T, Pedersen O, Polonsky KS, Bell GI: Mutations in the hepatocyte nuclear factor-1alpha gene in maturity-onset diabetes of the young (MODY3). Nature 1996;384:455–458.
12 Vaxillaire M, Boccio V, Philippi A, Vigouroux C, Terwilliger J, Passa P, Beckmann JS, Velho G, Lathrop GM, Froguel P: A gene for maturity-onset diabetes of the young (MODY) maps to chromosome 12q. Nat Genet 1995;9:418–423.
13 Froguel P, Zouali H, Vionnet N, Velho G, Vaxillaire M, Sun F, Lesage S, Stoffel M, Takeda J, Passa P: Familial hyperglycemia due to mutations in glucokinase. Definition of a subtype of diabetes mellitus. N Engl J Med 1993;328:697–702.
14 Frayling TM, Evans JC, Bulman MP, Pearson E, Allen L, Owen K, Bingham C, Hannemann M, Shepherd M, Ellard S, Hattersley AT: Beta-cell genes and diabetes: molecular and clinical characterization of mutations in transcription factors. Diabetes 2001; 50(suppl 1):S94–S100.
15 Lehto M, Tuomi T, Mahtani MM, Widen E, Forsblom C, Sarelin L, Gullstrom M, Isomaa B, Lehtovirta M, Hyrkko A, Kanninen T, Orho M, Manley S, Turner RC, Brettin T, Kirby A, Thomas J, Duyk G, Lander E, Taskinen MR, Groop L: Characterization of the MODY3 phenotype. Early-onset diabetes caused by an insulin secretion defect. J Clin Invest 1997;99:582–591.
16 Bellanne-Chantelot C, Chauveau D, Gautier JF, Dubois-Laforgue D, Clauin S, Beaufils S, Wilhelm JM, Boitard C, Noel LH, Velho G, Timsit J: Clinical spectrum associated with hepatocyte nuclear factor-1beta mutations. Ann Intern Med 2004;140: 510–517.
17 Ellard S, Bingham C, Jones K, Goodship J, Cole T, Van't Hoff W, Woolf A, Nicholls AJ, Hattersley AT: Hepatocyte nuclear factor 1-beta (HNF-1 beta): one gene – how many phenotypes? J Med Genet 2001; 38:S19.
18 Owen K, Hattersley AT: Maturity-onset diabetes of the young: from clinical description to molecular genetic characterization. Best Pract Res Clin Endocrinol Metab 2001;15:309–323.
19 Beckers D, Bellanne-Chantelot C, Maes M: Neonatal cholestatic jaundice as the first symptom of a mutation in the hepatocyte nuclear factor-1beta gene (HNF-1beta). J Pediatr 2007;150:313–314.
20 Bingham C, Ellard S, Cole TR, Jones KE, Allen LI, Goodship JA, Goodship TH, Bakalinova-Pugh D, Russell GI, Woolf AS, Nicholls AJ, Hattersley AT: Solitary functioning kidney and diverse genital tract malformations associated with hepatocyte nuclear factor-1beta mutations. Kidney Int 2002;61: 1243–1251.
21 Edghill EL, Bingham C, Slingerland AS, Minton JAL, Noordam C, Ellard S, Hattersley AT: Hepatocyte nuclear factor-1 beta mutations cause neonatal diabetes and intrauterine growth retardation: support for a critical role of HNF-1beta in human pancreatic development. Diabet Med 2006;23:1301–1306.
22 Maestro MA, Boj SF, Luco RF, Pierreux CE, Cabedo J, Servitja JM, German MS, Rousseau GG, Lemaigre FP, Ferrer J: Hnf6 and Tcf2 (MODY5) are linked in a gene network operating in a precursor cell domain of the embryonic pancreas. Hum Mol Genet 2003;12:3307–3314.
23 Barbacci E, Reber M, Ott MO, Breillat C, Huetz F, Cereghini S: Variant hepatocyte nuclear factor 1 is required for visceral endoderm specification. Development 1999;126:4795–4805.
24 Coffinier C, Thepot D, Babinet C, Yaniv M, Barra J: Essential role for the homeoprotein vHNF1/HNF1beta in visceral endoderm differentiation. Development 1999;126:4785–4794.
25 Haumaitre C, Barbacci E, Jenny M, Ott MO, Gradwohl G, Cereghini S: Lack of TCF2/vHNF1 in mice leads to pancreas agenesis. Proc Natl Acad Sci USA 2005;102:1490–1495.
26 Clotman F, Lannoy VJ, Reber M, Cereghini S, Cassiman D, Jacquemin P, Roskams T, Rousseau GG, Lemaigre FP: The onecut transcription factor HNF6 is required for normal development of the biliary tract. Development 2002;129:1819–1828.

27 Poll AV, Pierreux CE, Lokmane L, Haumaitre C, Achouri Y, Jacquemin P, Rousseau GG, Cereghini S, Lemaigre FP: A vHNF1/TCF2-HNF6 cascade regulates the transcription factor network that controls generation of pancreatic precursor cells. Diabetes 2006;55:61–69.
28 Haumaitre C, Fabre M, Cormier S, Baumann C, Delezoide AL, Cereghini S: Severe pancreas hypoplasia and multicystic renal dysplasia in two human fetuses carrying novel HNF1beta/MODY5 mutations. Hum Mol Genet 2006;15:2363–2375.
29 Yorifuji T, Kurokawa K, Mamada M, Imai T, Kawai M, Nishi Y, Shishido S, Hasegawa Y, Nakahata T: Neonatal diabetes mellitus and neonatal polycystic, dysplastic kidneys: phenotypically discordant recurrence of a mutation in the hepatocyte nuclear factor-1beta gene due to germline mosaicism. J Clin Endocrinol Metab 2004;89:2905–2908.
30 Stride A, Ellard S, Clark P, Shakespeare L, Salzmann M, Shepherd M, Hattersley AT: Beta-cell dysfunction, insulin sensitivity, and glycosuria precede diabetes in hepatocyte nuclear factor-1alpha mutation carriers. Diabetes Care 2005;28:1751–1756.
31 Tripathy D, Carlsson AL, Lehto M, Isomaa B, Tuomi T, Groop L: Insulin secretion and insulin sensitivity in diabetic subgroups: studies in the prediabetic and diabetic state. Diabetologia 2000;43:1476–1483.
32 Harries LW, Ellard S, Stride A, Morgan NG, Hattersley AT: Isomers of the TCF1 gene encoding hepatocyte nuclear factor-1 alpha show differential expression in the pancreas and define the relationship between mutation position and clinical phenotype in monogenic diabetes. Hum Mol Genet 2006;15:2216–2224.
33 Pontoglio M, Prie D, Cheret C, Doyen A, Leroy C, Froguel P, Velho G, Yaniv M, Friedlander G: HNF1-alpha controls renal glucose reabsorption in mouse and man. EMBO Rep 2000;1:359–365.
34 Cereghini S, Ott MO, Power S, Maury M: Expression patterns of vHNF1 and HNF1 homeoproteins in early postimplantation embryos suggest distinct and sequential developmental roles. Development 1992;116:783–797.
35 Nammo T, Yamagata K, Hamaoka R, Zhu Q, Akiyama TE, Gonzalez FJ, Miyagawa J, Matsuzawa Y: Expression profile of MODY3/HNF-1alpha protein in the developing mouse pancreas. Diabetologia 2002;45:1142–1153.
36 Lee YH, Sauer B, Gonzalez FJ: Laron dwarfism and non-insulin-dependent diabetes mellitus in the Hnf-1alpha knockout mouse. Mol Cell Biol 1998;18:3059–3068.
37 Pontoglio M, Barra J, Hadchouel M, Doyen A, Kress C, Bach JP, Babinet C, Yaniv M: Hepatocyte nuclear factor 1 inactivation results in hepatic dysfunction, phenylketonuria, and renal Fanconi syndrome. Cell 1996;84:575–585.
38 Pontoglio M, Sreenan S, Roe M, Pugh W, Ostrega D, Doyen A, Pick AJ, Baldwin A, Velho G, Froguel P, Levisetti M, Bonner-Weir S, Bell GI, Yaniv M, Polonsky KS: Defective insulin secretion in hepatocyte nuclear factor 1alpha-deficient mice. J Clin Invest 1998;101:2215–2222.
39 Dukes ID, Sreenan S, Roe MW, Levisetti M, Zhou YP, Ostrega D, Bell GI, Pontoglio M, Yaniv M, Philipson L, Polonsky KS: Defective pancreatic beta-cell glycolytic signaling in hepatocyte nuclear factor-1alpha-deficient mice. J Biol Chem 1998;273:24457–24464.
40 Parrizas M, Maestro MA, Boj SF, Paniagua A, Casamitjana R, Gomis R, Rivera R, Ferrer J: Hepatic nuclear factor 1-alpha directs nucleosomal hyperacetylation to its tissue-specific transcriptional targets. Mol Cell Biol 2001;21:3234–3243.
41 Shih DQ, Screenan S, Munoz KN, Philipson L, Pontoglio M, Yaniv M, Polonsky KS, Stoffel M: Loss of HNF-1alpha function in mice leads to abnormal expression of genes involved in pancreatic islet development and metabolism. Diabetes 2001;50:2472–2480.
42 Wang H, Antinozzi PA, Hagenfeldt KA, Maechler P, Wollheim CB: Molecular targets of a human HNF1alpha mutation responsible for pancreatic beta-cell dysfunction. EMBO J 2000;19:4257–4264.
43 Fukui K, Yang Q, Cao Y, Takahashi N, Hatakeyama H, Wang H, Wada J, Zhang Y, Marselli L, Nammo T, Yoneda K, Onishi M, Higashiyama S, Matsuzawa Y, Gonzalez FJ, Weir GC, Kasai H, Shimomura I, Miyagawa J, Wollheim CB, Yamagata K: The HNF-1 target collectrin controls insulin exocytosis by SNARE complex formation. Cell Metab 2005;2:373–384.
44 Akpinar P, Kuwajima S, Krutzfeldt J, Stoffel M: Tmem27: a cleaved and shed plasma membrane protein that stimulates pancreatic beta cell proliferation. Cell Metab 2005;2:385–397.
45 Odom DT, Zizlsperger N, Gordon DB, Bell GW, Rinaldi NJ, Murray HL, Volkert TL, Schreiber J, Rolfe PA, Gifford DK, Fraenkel E, Bell GI, Young RA: Control of pancreas and liver gene expression by HNF transcription factors. Science 2004;303:1378–1381.
46 Boj SF, Parrizas M, Maestro MA, Ferrer J: A transcription factor regulatory circuit in differentiated pancreatic cells. Proc Natl Acad Sci USA 2001;98:14481–14486.

47 Shepherd M, Hattersley AT: 'I don't feel like a diabetic any more': the impact of stopping insulin in patients with maturity-onset diabetes of the young following genetic testing. Clin Med 2004;4:144–147.
48 Pearson ER, Starkey BJ, Powell RJ, Gribble FM, Clark PM, Hattersley AT: Genetic cause of hyperglycaemia and response to treatment in diabetes. Lancet 2003;362:1275–1281.
49 Hattersley AT, Pearson ER: Minireview: pharmacogenetics and beyond: the interaction of therapeutic response, beta-cell physiology, and genetics in diabetes. Endocrinology 2006;147:2657–2663.
50 Luco RF, Maestro MA, del Pozo N, Philbrick WM, de la Ossa PP, Ferrer J: A conditional model reveals that induction of hepatocyte nuclear factor-1alpha in Hnf1alpha-null mutant beta-cells can activate silenced genes postnatally, whereas overexpression is deleterious. Diabetes 2006;55:2202–2211.
51 Hagenfeldt-Johansson KA, Herrera PL, Wang H, Gjinovci A, Ishihara H, Wollheim CB: Beta-cell-targeted expression of a dominant-negative hepatocyte nuclear factor-1 alpha induces a maturity-onset diabetes of the young (MODY)3-like phenotype in transgenic mice. Endocrinology 2001;142:5311–5320.
52 Efrat S, Linde S, Kofod H, Spector D, Delannoy M, Grant S, Hanahan D, Baekkeskov S: Beta-cell lines derived from transgenic mice expressing a hybrid insulin gene-oncogene. Proc Natl Acad Sci USA 1988;85:9037–9041.
53 Hanahan D: Heritable formation of pancreatic beta-cell tumours in transgenic mice expressing recombinant insulin/simian virus 40 oncogenes. Nature 1985;315:115–122.
54 Pearson ER, Pruhova S, Tack CJ, Johansen A, Castleden HAJ, Lumb PJ, Wierzbicki AS, Clark PM, Lebl J, Pedersen O, Ellard S, Hansen T, Hattersley AT: Molecular genetics and phenotypic characteristics of MODY caused by hepatocyte nuclear factor 4 alpha mutations in a large European collection. Diabetologia 2005;48:878–885.
55 Byrne MM, Sturis J, Fajans SS, Ortiz FJ, Stoltz A, Stoffel M, Smith MJ, Bell GI, Halter JB, Polonsky KS: Altered insulin secretory responses to glucose in subjects with a mutation in the MODY1 gene on chromosome 20. Diabetes 1995;44:699–704.
56 Byrne MM, Sturis J, Menzel S, Yamagata K, Fajans SS, Dronsfield MJ, Bain SC, Hattersley AT, Velho G, Froguel P, Bell GI, Polonsky KS: Altered insulin secretory responses to glucose in diabetic and nondiabetic subjects with mutations in the diabetes susceptibility gene MODY3 on chromosome 12. Diabetes 1996;45:1503–1510.
57 Gloyn AL, Ellard S, Shepherd M, Howell RT, Parry EM, Jefferson A, Levy ER, Hattersley AT: Maturity-onset diabetes of the young caused by a balanced translocation where the 20q12 break point results in disruption upstream of the coding region of hepatocyte nuclear factor-4alpha (HNF4A) gene. Diabetes 2002;51:2329–2333.
58 Ferrer J: A genetic switch in pancreatic beta-cells: implications for differentiation and haploinsufficiency. Diabetes 2002;51:2355–2362.
59 Hansen SK, Parrizas M, Jensen ML, Pruhova S, Ek J, Boj SF, Johansen A, Maestro MA, Rivera F, Eiberg H, Andel M, Lebl J, Pedersen O, Ferrer J, Hansen T: Genetic evidence that HNF-1alpha-dependent transcriptional control of HNF-4alpha is essential for human pancreatic beta cell function. J Clin Invest 2002;110:827–833.
60 Servitja JM, Ferrer J: Transcriptional networks controlling pancreatic development and beta cell function. Diabetologia 2004;47:597–613.
61 Thomas H, Jaschkowitz K, Bulman M, Frayling TM, Mitchell SM, Roosen S, Lingott-Frieg A, Tack CJ, Ellard S, Ryffel GU, Hattersley AT: A distant upstream promoter of the HNF-4alpha gene connects the transcription factors involved in maturity-onset diabetes of the young. Hum Mol Genet 2001;10: 2089–2097.
62 Kuo CJ, Conley PB, Chen L, Sladek FM, Darnell JE Jr, Crabtree GR: A transcriptional hierarchy involved in mammalian cell-type specification. Nature 1992;355:457–461.
63 Kyrmizi I, Hatzis P, Katrakili N, Tronche F, Gonzalez FJ, Talianidis I: Plasticity and expanding complexity of the hepatic transcription factor network during liver development. Genes Dev 2006;20: 2293–2305.
64 Tian JM, Schibler U: Tissue-specific expression of the gene encoding hepatocyte nuclear factor 1 may involve hepatocyte nuclear factor 4. Genes Dev 1991;5:2225–2234.
65 Wang H, Maechler P, Antinozzi PA, Hagenfeldt KA, Wollheim CB: Hepatocyte nuclear factor 4alpha regulates the expression of pancreatic beta-cell genes implicated in glucose metabolism and nutrient-induced insulin secretion. J Biol Chem 2000;275:35953–35959.
66 Gupta RK, Vatamaniuk MZ, Lee CS, Flaschen RC, Fulmer JT, Matschinsky FM, Duncan SA, Kaestner KH: The MODY1 gene HNF-4alpha regulates selected genes involved in insulin secretion. J Clin Invest 2005;115:1006–1015.

67 Miura A, Yamagata K, Kakei M, Hatakeyama H, Takahashi N, Fukui K, Nammo T, Yoneda K, Inoue Y, Sladek FM, Magnuson MA, Kasai H, Miyagawa J, Gonzalez FJ, Shimomura I: Hepatocyte nuclear factor-4alpha is essential for glucose-stimulated insulin secretion by pancreatic beta-cells. J Biol Chem 2006;281:5246–5257.

68 Pearson E, Steele A, Stals K, Ellard S, Barrett T, Hattersley A, Shield J: HNF-4a mutations cause fetal hyperinsulinaemia, macrosomia and transient neonatal hypoglycaemia. Horm Res 2006;65:18.

69 Eeckhoute J, Moerman E, Bouckenooghe T, Lukoviak B, Pattou F, Formstecher P, Kerr-Conte J, Vandewalle B, Laine B: Hepatocyte nuclear factor 4 alpha isoforms originated from the P1 promoter are expressed in human pancreatic beta-cells and exhibit stronger transcriptional potentials than P2 promoter-driven isoforms. Endocrinology 2003; 144:1686–1694

70 Ktistaki E, Talianidis I: Modulation of hepatic gene expression by hepatocyte nuclear factor 1. Science 1997;277:109–112.

71 Chen WS, Manova K, Weinstein DC, Duncan SA, Plump AS, Prezioso VR, Bachvarova RF, Darnell JE Jr: Disruption of the HNF-4 gene, expressed in visceral endoderm leads to cell death in embryonic ectoderm and impaired gastrulation of mouse embryos. Genes Dev 1994;8:2466–2477.

72 Gupta RK, Gao N, Gorski RK, White P, Hardy OT, Rafiq K, Brestelli JE, Chen G, Stoeckert CJ Jr, Kaestner KH: Expansion of adult beta-cell mass in response to increased metabolic demand is dependent on HNF-4alpha. Genes Dev 2007;21:756–769.

Dr. Jorge Ferrer
Genomic Programming of Beta Cells Laboratory
Institut d'Investigacions Biomèdiques August Pi i Sunyer
Endocrinology, Hospital Clínic de Barcelona
Villarroel 170, ES–08036 Barcelona (Spain)
Tel. +34 93 227 5400, ext. 3028, Fax +34 93 451 6638, E-Mail jferrer@clinic.ub.es

Shield JPH, Scharfmann R (eds): Development of the Pancreas and Neonatal Diabetes.
Endocr Dev. Basel, Karger, 2007, vol 12, pp 46–54

In vivo and in vitro Techniques to Study Pancreas Development and Islet Cell Function

Bertrand Duvillié · Mylène Heinis · Volodymyr Stetsyuk
INSERM U845, Necker Hospital, Faculty of Medicine, University Paris-Descartes, Paris, France

Abstract
Over the last decades, pancreas development has been widely investigated. Understanding the mechanisms that control β-cell development should allow progress towards the regeneration of these cells in humans. Particularly, it is well established that inductive signals from the mesenchyme play an essential role in the proliferation of precursor cells. In the present review, we focused on the roles of fibroblast growth factors (FGFs) in pancreas development. Improvements of the in vivo and in vitro techniques were used to define the function of FGF10. Experiments on FGF10 knockout mice showed that FGF10 is required for the proliferation of precursor cells and the pancreas development. Several laboratories used different in vitro techniques to study the effect of FGF10 on β-cell differentiation. These methods of investigation are described here. In our experiments, pancreases were placed at the air-liquid interface to define the precise mechanism of action of FGF10. We showed that FGF10 positively regulates the β-cell mass by increasing the proliferation of the early precursors and by extending the window of expression of the endocrine precursor marker Ngn3. These data are compared with studies performed with other culture systems. Finally, the role of other FGFs is discussed.

Diabetes mellitus arises from an inadequate mass of β-cells leading to hyperglycemia and a number of complications. Given the crucial role of β-cells to regulate glycemia, numerous studies have investigated the factors that control islet cell development. Such studies are essential to help develop strategies for a cell-based approach towards the repopulation of the endocrine pancreas for the treatment of type 1 diabetes.

The embryonic gut of vertebrates consists of the endodermal epithelium and surrounding mesenchyme. Although the gut is initially a simple tube, it becomes divided anteroposteriorly into various organs [1]. The pancreas originates from two evaginations of the endodermal primitive gut tube at 20–22 somite stages in the mouse.

These regions are found immediately posterior to the stomach [2, 3]. These two pancreatic buds, dorsal and ventral, will fuse later during development forming a unique organ. The embryonic pancreas contains an epithelium surrounded by mesenchyme. The early epithelial cells express the transcription factor pancreatic duodenal homeobox-1 (Pdx1). In the mature pancreas, its expression is restricted to the differentiated β-cells [4]. In the mouse, the disruption of Pdx1 leads to pancreatic agenesis [5]. In humans, the deletion of a single nucleotide also causes absence of pancreas development [6]. These data indicate that Pdx1 is necessary for pancreas morphogenesis and differentiation. This transcription factor is also a useful marker to detect the pancreatic progenitors.

Epithelio-mesenchymal interactions have been studied since the early 1960s. Golosow and Grobstein [7] performed in vitro experiments using embryonic day 11 (E11) mouse pancreatic rudiments. Their data indicated that the mesenchyme was necessary for pancreas development. Indeed, epithelia cultured with the surrounding mesenchyme developed but such a development did not take place when they were cultured in the absence of their mesenchyme. Moreover, epithelia recombined with heterogeneous mesenchymes underwent morphogenesis resembling the intact pancreases [7]. Many recent studies also show that the pancreatic mesenchyme is important to guide the exocrine and endocrine differentiation events [8–14]. Particularly, the pancreas appears to be a unique model to study the balance between the profileration of the precursor cells and their differentiation. In our laboratory, we developed several in vivo and in vitro approaches to investigate the role of the fibroblast growth factors (FGFs) in pancreas development. The FGF family contains 23 members. We focused on FGF10 because it is one of the growth factors expressed in the pancreas during development. Its expression occurs during early development and is restricted to the mesenchyme [15]. The receptor of FGF10, FGFr2IIIb, is expressed in the epithelial cells [15]. These data indicate that FGF10 finds target cells among the precursor cells. The methods to investigate the role of FGFs in pancreas development will be presented first, and then the roles of FGF10 will be reviewed.

Methods

In vivo Techniques

Generation of Knockout Mice

The production of knockout animals is based on the ability of embryonic stem cells (ES cells) to generate all types of tissues. ES cells are multipotent. Indeed, they are able to differentiate into germ cells when they are incorporated in a host mouse. Once ES cells are mutated, they are introduced in recipient mice. These chimeric mice are intercrossed and knockout animals are obtained in their offspring.

The first step to generate knockout animals is to derive ES cells from the inner cell mass of a blastocyst. These cells are cultured and electroporated with targeting vector DNA containing a neomycin resistance gene and a thymidine kinase gene. The neomycin gene permits a positive selection of the clones using a drug, G418, and the thymidine kinase gene allows a negative selection of the recombinant events using a drug, ganciclovir. Indeed, when the targeting vector is inserted by homologous recombination at the correct locus, the thymidine kinase gene giving the sensitivity to ganciclovir is eliminated. The second step is to introduce the recombinated ES cells into a host blastocyst using a microinjection system. Finally, the third step is to place the chimeric blastocyst in the uterus of a foster mother. The resulting chimeric animals will transmit the mutation to their offspring.

In vitro Techniques

Animals

Pregnant Wistar rats were purchased from the Janvier breeding center (CERJ, Le Genest, France). The first day post coitum was taken as E0.5. The animals had free access to food pellets and water. Pregnant female rats at 13.5 days of gestation were sacrificed by CO_2 asphyxiation, according to the guidelines of the French Animal Care Committee.

Dissection of Pancreatic Rudiments

The embryos were harvested on E13.5. The dorsal pancreatic bud was dissected as described previously [16]. Briefly, the stomach, the pancreas, and a small portion of the intestine were dissected together; then, either the pancreatic primordium was dissected or the mesenchyme was separated from the pancreatic epithelium as follows: the digestive tract was incubated with 0.5 mg/ml collagenase A (Roche, Meylan, France) at 37°C for 20 min then washed several times with Hank's balanced salt solution (Invitrogen, Cergy-Pontoise, France) at 4°C, and the epithelium was mechanically separated from the surrounding mesenchyme using needles on 0.25% agar, 25% Hank's balanced salt solution, and 75% RPMI (Gibco, Cergy-Pontoise, France) gel in a Petri dish.

Organ Culture

Dorsal pancreatic rudiments with or without their mesenchyme were laid on Millicell culture plate inserts (Millipore, Molsheim, France) in 35-mm sterile Petri dishes containing 2 ml of RPMI-1640 (Invitrogen) supplemented with penicillin (100 U/ml), streptomycin (100 μg/ml), Hepes (10 mmol/l), L-glutamine (2 mmol/l), nonessential amino acids (×1, Gibco), and 10% heat-inactivated calf serum (Hyclone, Logan, Utah, USA). Under such culture conditions, the explants grew at the air-medium interface. Cultures were maintained at 37°C in humidified 95% air/5% CO_2. The medium was changed every other day.

Recombinant human FGF10 (R&D Systems, Lille, France) was used at a concentration of 50 ng/ml in the presence of heparin (Sigma, Saint-Quentin-Fallavier, France) at a concentration of 50 μg/ml. To ensure labeling of cells in the S phase, bromodeoxyuridine (BrdU; 10 μM) was added to the culture medium. At the end of the culture period, the pancreatic rudiments were photographed and fixed.

Analysis of the Tissues by Immunohistochemistry

Tissues were fixed in 10% formalin, pre-embedded in agarose gel [4% of type VII low-gelling-temperature agarose (Sigma, Saint-Quentin-Fallavier, France)], and embedded in paraffin. Sections (4 μm thick) were collected and processed for immunohistochemistry, as described previously [16, 17]. To detect the precursor cells, rabbit anti-PDX1 antibody (1/1,000) was used. To visualize and measure the cells that proliferate, mouse anti-BrdU (Amersham, Uppsala, Sweden, 1/2) [17] was used. To detect β-cell development, the antibodies were used at the following dilutions: mouse anti-human insulin (Sigma, 1/2,000), rabbit anti-insulin (Diasorin, Antony, France,

1/2,000). The fluorescent secondary antibodies were fluorescein isothiocyanate anti-rabbit antibody (Jackson Immunoresearch, USA, 1/200), Texas red anti-mouse antibody (Jackson, 1/200) and Alexa fluor anti-rabbit antibody (Biogenex, San Ramon, USA, 1/400). Nuclei were labeled using Hoechst. Photographs were taken using a fluorescence microscope (Leica, Leitz DMRB) and digitized using a Hamamatsu (Middlesex, N.J., USA) C5810 cooled 3CCD camera. No signals were observed when the first antibodies were omitted.

In situ Hybridization
Tissues were fixed at 4°C in 4% paraformaldehyde in phosphate-buffered saline, cryoprotected in 15% sucrose/phosphate-buffered saline at 4°C overnight, embedded in 15% sucrose/7.5% gelatin in phosphate-buffered saline, and frozen at –50°C in isopentane. Cryosections 14 μm in thickness were prepared. The *Ngn3* probe (726 bp) was prepared as previously described [18]. Plasmids were linearized and used as templates for synthesizing sense or antisense riboprobes using T7 or SP6 RNA polymerase (Roche), in the presence of digoxigenin-UTP (Roche Diagnostic). In situ hybridization was done as previously described [19], and colorimetric revelation was performed with 5-bromo-4-chloro-3-indolyl phosphate (Promega, Charbonnières, France) and nitroblue tetrazolium (Roche) to obtain a blue precipitate. Photographs were digitized using a Hamamatsu C5810 cooled 3CCD camera. No signal was obtained when a sense riboprobe was used.

Results and Discussion

Analysis of the Pancreatic Development in FGF10 Knockout Mice

In situ hybridization revealed that FGF10 expression starts at E9.5 in the area of the gut tube where the pancreas forms in the mouse. Next its expression is restricted to the pancreatic mesenchyme that surrounds the epithelial buds at E10.5 and E11.5 and disappears later at E12.5 [15]. The receptor of FGF10, FGFR2IIIb, is expressed in the pancreatic epithelium [20, 21], suggesting that FGF10 produced by the mesenchyme provides instructive signals to the epithelium. The production of FGF10$^{-/-}$ mutant mice has previously been described [22]. In the mutant embryos at E17.5, the gastrointestinal tract was normal but the pancreas and the stomach were dramatically reduced in size. The developed tissue contained acinar cells but was devoid of islets [15]. One hypothesis was a defect of the pool of progenitors. In order to examine the early progenitors, expression of Pdx1, a marker of these cells, was investigated by immunohistochemistry and in situ hybridization. Indeed, *Pdx1* expression occurs when the endoderm is committed to a pancreatic fate and its expression remains present in all epithelial cells [23–25]. Expression of *Pdx1* was detected at E10.5 and extended later in wild-type embryos. On the other hand, *Pdx1* expression was significantly reduced in FGF10$^{-/-}$ embryos [15]. To determine the mechanism by which the pool of precursor cells was depleted, their proliferation was quantified after BrdU incorporation. BrdU incorporation is an accurate method to measure cell proliferation because it is a direct assay of DNA synthesis [26]. BrdU is a halogenated derivative of thymidine that is incorporated into DNA only in the S phase of the cell cycle. It can be detected by immunohistochemistry using monoclonal antibodies In the wild-type pancreas, a high percentage of precursor cells were proliferating. In contrast, very rare *Pdx1*-positive cells had incorporated BrdU in the FGF10$^{-/-}$ embryos. This suggests that the reduced pancreas in FGF10$^{-/-}$ mutant mice is likely caused by the defect of proliferation of the *Pdx1*-positive precursor cells [15].

One other possibility might have been the accelerated differentiation of the precursor cells into endocrine cells. Such a phenotype has been described in mice lacking *Hes1* [27]. Hes1 is a member of the hairy and enhancer of split (Hes) proteins and is a direct target of the activated Notch receptor. Several studies have pointed out the role of Notch-mediated control of the pancreatic fate determination via control of *Ngn3* [28]. The *Hes1* mutant mice displayed a defect of pancreas development. This phenotype resulted from the depletion of the precursor cells caused by accelerated differentiation of the endocrine cells [27]. In FGF10$^{-/-}$ mice, no precocious differentiation of endocrine cells was detected, and consequently we can exclude this hypothesis.

Analysis of the Role of FGF10 Using in vitro Techniques

In the in vivo study described above, the data, using a loss-of-function approach, show that FGF10 directly and positively controls the mass of β-cells. On the other hand, other transgenic animals, using a gain-of-function strategy, suggested that FGF10 could inhibit β-cell differentiation [29, 30]. Indeed, when persistent FGF10 expression driven by the Pdx1 promoter was induced in transgenic mice, hyperplasia of the pancreas was detected and endocrine differentiation was arrested [29]. This result was unexpected. One possibility could be that the phenotype of the pPdx1-FGF10 mice is due to the early expression of *Pdx1*. Indeed, *Pdx1* is normally expressed before the mesenchyme condenses and the pPdx1-FGF10 transgene could therefore induce nonphysiological effects. In order to determine the exact mechanism of FGF10 effect, we next used culture experiments. The pancreases from E13.5 rat embryos were dissected as described previously [12, 13, 17] and as presented in figure 1. The pancreases were cultured on filters at the air-liquid interface (fig. 2). The role of the mesenchyme was first analyzed. To this end, pancreases were depleted of their mesenchyme (see fig. 3 for the dissection) and cultured at the air-liquid interface. They were compared to whole pancreases cultured in the same conditions. In the presence of the mesenchyme, the mass of β-cells that differentiated was significantly increased as compared to epithelia cultured alone. This was not due to induction of the proliferation of β-cells by the mesenchyme [13]. The proliferation of the early progenitors was quantified by measuring BrdU incorporation. BrdU was added during the last hour of culture and immunohistochemistry with anti-BrdU and anti-Pdx1 was performed. After 1 day of culture with the mesenchyme, the percentage of proliferating precursor cells was 8 times higher than without the mesenchyme. Consequently, the number of *Ngn3*-positive endocrine precursors was increased and the time of *Ngn3*

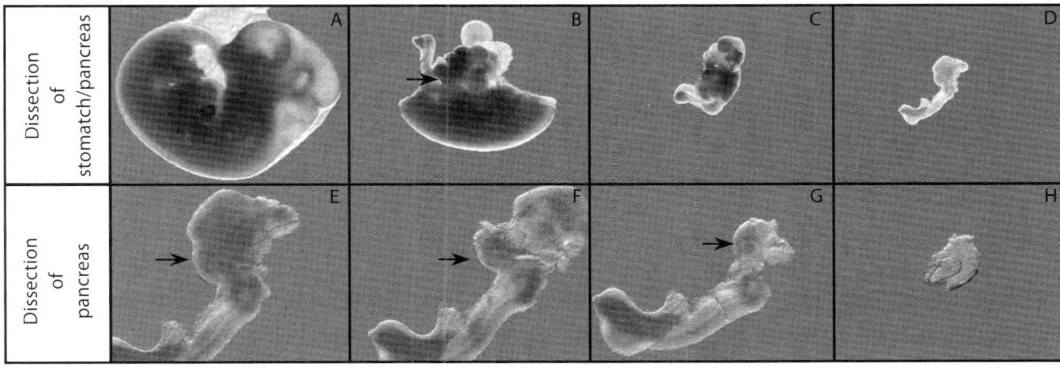

Fig. 1. A–C Dissection of the block of internal organs containing the stomach, intestine and duodenum. **E–H** Dissection of the pancreas. **A** Rat embryos are harvested at E13.5. **B** The head and the tail are removed. **C** The internal organs containing the lung, liver, stomach, pancreas and intestine are harvested. **D** The block of stomach-pancreas-intestine is isolated. **E** The arrow indicates the embryonic pancreas. **F** The stomach is separated from the pancreas (arrow). **G** The pancreas (arrow) is separated from the intestine. **H** The pancreas containing the epithelium and mesenchyme is isolated.

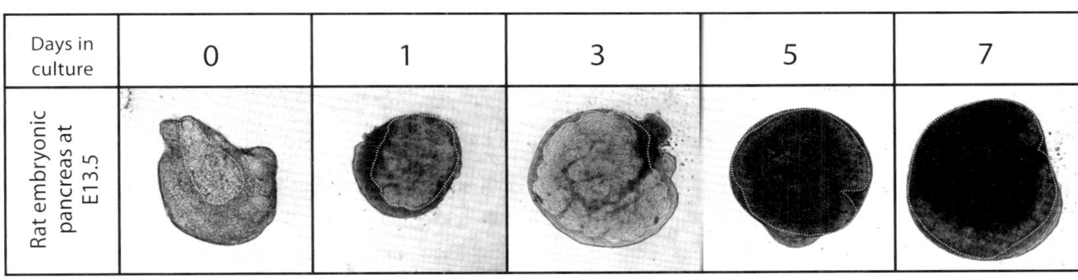

Fig. 2. Culture of rat embryonic pancreases at the air-liquid interface for 0, 1, 3, 5, and 7 days. The pancreatic epithelium grows and spreads within the surrounding mesenchyme.

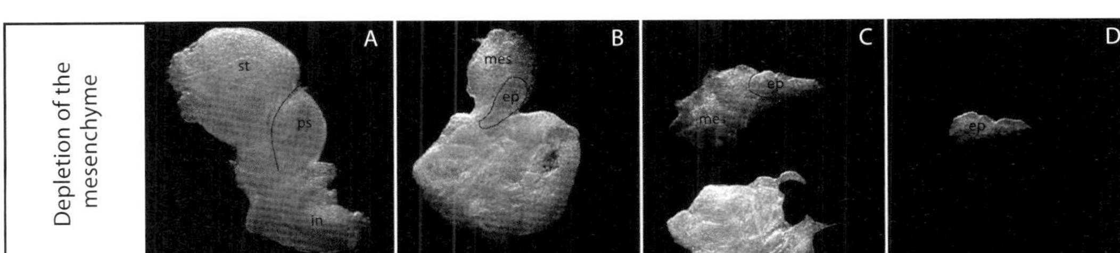

Fig. 3. Dissection of the pancreatic epithelium. **A** Block of the stomach (st), pancreas (ps), and intestine (in) previously digested by collagenase I. **B** The embryonic pancreas containing epithelium (ep) and mesenchyme (mes) is separated from the rest of the tissue. **C** The pancreas is isolated and the mesenchyme is separated from the epithelium with needles. **D** Isolated epithelium.

expression was extended [13]. The same effects were found when FGF10 was added to the culture of epithelia devoid of the mesenchyme. Altogether, these data demonstrate that FGF10 positively regulates the β-cell mass by inducing proliferation of the progenitor cells [13].

Study of the Role of FGF10 Using Other in vitro Techniques

Recently, Miralles et al. [31] have used another culture system to study the effect of FGF10 on β-cell development. Indeed, mouse embryonic epithelia at E10.5 were placed within a matrix of growth-factor-reduced Matrigel in the presence or absence of FGF10. In such conditions, the proliferation of the precursors was induced by FGF10 but the differentiation of the β-cells was inhibited. Experimental evidences indicated that the effect of FGF10 on the self-renewal of the progenitors was dependent on active Notch signaling [31]. In order to explain the discrepancy between these results with E10.5 mouse pancreases and our data with E13.5 rat pancreases, we propose that the stage of the pancreases used for these experiments may determine its competence to respond to FGF10. Indeed, at E10.5 in the mouse, the embryonic pancreas is less developed than at E13.5 in the rat. We might expect that at E10.5 in the mouse, addition of FGF10 could affect the differentiation program leading to a different phenotype than using E13.5 pancreases. In order to determine the physiological relevance of our studies, we analyzed the expression of several genes including *Nkx6.2, Ngn3, Pax4, Pcsk1* and *Pcsk22* in E13.5 pancreases cultured on a filter. We found that their expression patterns in vitro were similar to the in vivo condition [13]. Therefore, the culture of E13.5 rat embryonic pancreas at the air-liquid interface appears to be representative of a physiological development.

Role of FGF7

The growth factor FGF7 is another ligand of FGFR2IIIb [32]. The effect of the activation of FGFR2IIIb by FGF7 has been monitored in vitro using a culture in a three-dimensional collagen gel. In this culture system, β-cells differentiate when the epithelium is grown without but not with the mesenchyme [20]. Moreover, the mesenchyme induced the proliferation of the epithelial precursor cells but repressed endocrine differentiation. This effect was mimicked by FGF7 when it was added to pancreatic epithelium cultures. When pancreatic epithelia were grown with FGF7, epithelial cell proliferation occurred in a dose-dependent manner and endocrine development was inhibited [33]. The epithelial cells that proliferated when FGF7 was added were endocrine precursors as they differentiated en masse into β-cells on FGF7 removal [33]. These data demonstrate that FGFs can be used to facilitate the expansion of the endocrine progenitors in vitro.

Conclusion

Altogether, the presented data show that in vivo and in vitro techniques are complementary strategies to understand the role of the mesenchyme and particularly of FGF10 in pancreas development. The culture of the pancreas at the air-liquid interface is a very useful tool to study pancreas development as the genes determining the cell lineages are expressed similarly to in vivo. The studies reviewed here indicate that the proliferation of progenitors can be induced in vitro. Moreover, recent data have shown that FGF7 and FGF10 can also activate the proliferation of human pancreatic progenitors in vitro [34]. This approach should constitute a step towards the production of human β-cells and facilitate a cell therapy of type 1 diabetes.

References

1 Fukuda K, Sakamoto N, Narita T, et al: Application of efficient and specific gene transfer systems and organ culture techniques for the elucidation of mechanisms of epithelial-mesenchymal interaction in the developing gut. Dev Growth Differ 2000; 42:207–211.

2 Pictet RL, Clark WR, Williams RH, Rutter WJ: An ultrastructural analysis of the developing embryonic pancreas Dev Biol 1972;29:436–467.

3 Wessells NK, Cohen JH: The influence of collagen and embryo extract on the development of pancreatic epithelium. Exp Cell Res 1966;43:680–684.

4 Ohlsson H, Karlsson K, Edlund T: IPF1, a homeodomain-containing transactivator of the insulin gene. EMBO J 1993;12:4251–4259.

5 Offield MF, Jetton TL, Labosky PA, et al: PDX-1 is required for pancreatic outgrowth and differentiation of the rostral duodenum. Development 1996; 122:983–995.

6 Stoffers DA, Zinkin NT, Stanojevic V, Clarke WL, Habener JF: Pancreatic agenesis attributable to a single nucleotide deletion in the human IPF1 gene coding sequence. Nat Genet 1997;15:106–110.

7 Golosow N, Grobstein C: Epitheliomesenchymal interaction in pancreatic morphogenesis. Dev Biol 1962;4:242–255.

8 Li Z, Manna P, Kobayashi H, et al: Multifaceted pancreatic mesenchymal control of epithelial lineage selection. Dev Biol 2004;269:252–263.

9 Levine S, Pictet R, Rutter WJ: Control of cell proliferation and cytodifferentiation by a factor reacting with the cell surface. Nat New Biol 1973;246:49–52.

10 Gittes GK, Galante PE, Hanahan D, Rutter WJ, Debase HT: Lineage-specific morphogenesis in the developing pancreas: role of mesenchymal factors. Development 1996;122:439–447.

11 Miralles F, Serup P, Cluzeaud F, Vandewalle A, Czernichow P, Scharfmann R: Characterization of beta cells developed in vitro from rat embryonic pancreatic epithelium. Dev Dyn 1999;214:116–126.

12 Duvillie B, Attali M, Bounacer A, Ravassard P, Basmaciogullari A, Scharfmann R: The mesenchyme controls the timing of pancreatic beta-cell differentiation. Diabetes 2006;55:582–589.

13 Attali M, Stetsyuk V, Basmaciogullari A, et al: Control of beta-cell differentiation by the pancreatic mesenchyme. Diabetes 2007;56:1248–1258.

14 Rutter WJ: The development of the endocrine and exocrine pancreas. Monogr Pathol 1980;21:30–38.

15 Bhushan A, Itoh N, Kato S, et al: Fgf10 is essential for maintaining the proliferative capacity of epithelial progenitor cells during early pancreatic organogenesis. Development 2001;128:5109–5117.

16 Miralles F, Czernichow P, Scharfmann R: Follistatin regulates the relative proportions of endocrine versus exocrine tissue during pancreatic development. Development 1998;125:1017–1024.

17 Duvillie B, Attali M, Aiello V, Quemeneur E, Scharfmann R: Label-retaining cells in the rat pancreas: location and differentiation potential in vitro. Diabetes 2003;52:2035–2042.

18 Ravassard P, Chatail F, Mallet J, Icard-Liepkalns C: Relax, a novel rat bHLH transcriptional regulator transiently expressed in the ventricular proliferating zone of the developing central nervous system. J Neurosci Res 1997;48:146–158.

19 Herzog E, Bellenchi GC, Gras C, et al: The existence of a second vesicular glutamate transporter specifies subpopulations of glutamatergic neurons. J Neurosci 2001;21:RC181.

20 Miralles F, Czernichow P, Ozaki K, Itoh N, Scharfmann R: Signaling through fibroblast growth factor receptor 2b plays a key role in the development of the exocrine pancreas. Proc Natl Acad Sci USA 1999;96:6267–6272.
21 Finch PW, Cunha GR, Rubin JS, Wong J, Ron D: Pattern of keratinocyte growth factor and keratinocyte growth factor receptor expression during mouse fetal development suggests a role in mediating morphogenetic mesenchymal-epithelial interactions. Dev Dyn 1995;203:223–240.
22 Sekine K, Ohuchi H, Fujiwara M, et al: Fgf10 is essential for limb and lung formation. Nat Genet 1999;21:138–141.
23 Ahlgren U, Jonsson J, Edlund H: The morphogenesis of the pancreatic mesenchyme is uncoupled from that of the pancreatic epithelium in IPF1/PDX1-deficient mice. Development 1996;122:1409–1416.
24 Guz Y, Montminy MR, Stein R, et al: Expression of murine STF-1, a putative insulin gene transcription factor, in beta cells of pancreas, duodenal epithelium and pancreatic exocrine and endocrine progenitors during ontogeny. Development 1995;121:11–18.
25 Jonsson J, Carlsson L, Edlund T, Edlund H: Insulin-promoter-factor 1 is required for pancreas development in mice. Nature 1994;371:606–609.
26 Dolbeare F: Bromodeoxyuridine: a diagnostic tool in biology and medicine. 2. Oncology, chemotherapy and carcinogenesis. Histochem J 1995;27:923–964.
27 Jensen J, Pedersen EE, Galante P, et al: Control of endodermal endocrine development by Hes-1. Nat Genet 2000;24:36–44.
28 Hald J, Hjorth JP, German MS, Madsen OD, Serup P, Jensen J: Activated Notch1 prevents differentiation of pancreatic acinar cells and attenuate endocrine development. Dev Biol 2003;260:426–437.
29 Hart A, Papadopoulou S, Edlund H: Fgf10 maintains notch activation, stimulates proliferation, and blocks differentiation of pancreatic epithelial cells. Dev Dyn 2003;228:185–193.
30 Norgaard GA, Jensen JN, Jensen J: FGF10 signaling maintains the pancreatic progenitor cell state revealing a novel role of Notch in organ development. Dev Biol 2003;264:323–338.
31 Miralles F, Lamotte L, Couton D, Joshi RL: Interplay between FGF10 and Notch signalling is required for the self-renewal of pancreatic progenitors. Int J Dev Biol 2006;50:17–26.
32 Ornitz DM, Xu J, Colvin JS, et al: Receptor specificity of the fibroblast growth factor family. J Biol Chem 1996;271:15292–15297.
33 Elghazi L, Cras-Meneur C, Czernichow P, Scharfmann R: Role for FGFR2IIIb-mediated signals in controlling pancreatic endocrine progenitor cell proliferation. Proc Natl Acad Sci USA 2002;99:3884–3889.
34 Ye F, Duvillie B, Scharfmann R: Fibroblast growth factors 7 and 10 are expressed in the human embryonic pancreatic mesenchyme and promote the proliferation of embryonic pancreatic epithelial cells. Diabetologia 2005;48:277–281.

Dr. Bertrand Duvillié
INSERM U845, Faculté Necker
156, rue de Vaugirard, FR–75015 Paris (France)
Tel. +33 1 40 61 55 65, Fax +33 1 43 06 04 43, E-Mail duvillie@necker.fr

Shield JPH, Scharfmann R (eds): Development of the Pancreas and Neonatal Diabetes.
Endocr Dev. Basel, Karger, 2007, vol 12, pp 55–66

Functional Imaging of the Pancreas: The Role of [^{18}F]Fluoro-L-DOPA PET in the Diagnosis of Hyperinsulinism of Infancy

Maria-João Ribeiro[a] · Nathalie Boddaert[b] · Thierry Delzescaux[a] · Vassili Valayannopoulos[b] · Christine Bellanné-Chartelot[b] · Francis Jaubert[b] · Virginie Verkarre[b] · Claire Nihoul-Fékété[b] · Francis Brunelle[b] · Pascale De Lonlay[b]

[a]Life Sciences Division, Biomedical Imaging Institute, Frédéric Joliot Hospital, CEA, Orsay, and
[b]Departments of Radiology, Pediatrics, Surgery and Pathology, Necker-Enfants Malades Hospital, AP-HP, Paris, France

Abstract

Congenital hyperinsulinism (HI) of infancy, the most frequent cause of hypoglycaemia in young children, is a neuro-endocrine disease secondary to either focal adenomatous hyperplasia or a diffuse abnormal pancreatic insulin secretion. This inappropriate secretion of insulin induces severe hypoglycaemias that require aggressive treatment to prevent the high risk of irreversible brain damage. Focal and diffuse forms of HI share a similar clinical presentation, but their treatment is dramatically different. Selective surgical resection can cure focal HI whilst diffuse forms require near-total pancreatectomy if resistant to medical treatment. Until recently, preoperative differential diagnosis was based on pancreatic venous sampling, an invasive method, technically difficult to perform, which requires general anaesthesia. The pancreas is one of the most heavily innervated peripheral organs in the body, and its functional imaging with positron emission tomography (PET) is difficult to perform, in part because of the vast number of physiological roles and cell types that characterize this organ. However, HI, as all neuro-endocrine diseases, is notable for the ability to take up amine precursors and to convert them into biogenic amines. Therefore, we have evaluated the use of PET with [^{18}F]fluoro-L-DOPA, a precursor of catecholamines, to image the pancreas and distinguish focal from diffuse HI.

Congenital hyperinsulinism (HI), previously named persistent hyperinsulinaemic hypoglycaemia, with a permanent increase in insulin secretion is the most important cause of recurrent and profound hypoglycaemia in early infancy with an incidence of 1:50,000 live births [1–3]. Prompt recognition and correction of hypoglycaemia are necessary to prevent the high risk of permanent neurological complications [4].

Diagnosis of HI is based on the development of hypoglycaemia during fasting and postprandially (plasma glucose concentration <3 mmol/l) with hyperinsulinaemia (plasma insulin concentration >10 μU/ml, 60 pmol/l) without ketone bodies, and with an increase in plasma concentration (>5 mmol/l) in response to administration of glucagon [5–8].

Pharmacological control of HI commonly involves therapy with diazoxide with or without octreotide and/or nifedipine [9–11], which inhibit insulin secretion. In addition, frequent feedings with a carbohydrate-enriched diet are utilized. However, frequently this treatment is not effective and pancreatectomy is the only option for patients resistant to treatment [5, 12]. HI can be related at least to two different histopathological forms based on different molecular entities and despite an indistinguishable clinical presentation: focal and diffuse forms [1, 2, 13–17]. Focal HI is characterized by pathological pancreatic β-cells gathered in focal adenomatous hyperplasia always limited to a small area with a 2.5- to 7.5-mm diameter. The focal form is composed of either ramified or branched areas of clear endocrine cells surrounded frequently by a thin rim of acini at the periphery; they can involve multiple adjacent lobules with mainly abnormal β-cells occupying their centre. Sometimes it may appear as a polyp at the pancreas surface which is easy to find for the surgeon or it may be deeper inside the pancreas with consequential problems in locating and identifying safe margins to avoid postoperative relapse due to incomplete removal. More rarely the abnormal foci can be extrapancreatic. The endocrine cells themselves have an abundant cytoplasm with nuclei far apart of irregular size and from time to time a very big oversized nucleus of irregular angulated shape which is more than 3–4 times the size of nearby acinic nuclei taken as the control [18]. Conversely, in diffuse HI there is abnormal insulin secretion by all pancreatic β-cells, with disseminated β-cells displaying enlarged abnormal nuclei [3, 18]. About 10% of HI cases are clinically atypical and cannot be classified, having an unknown molecular basis and histopathological form; even if the pattern of pancreas involvement is of the diffuse type, only one area might be involved corresponding to half of the pancreas [19]. The distinction between the two major forms of HI is crucial since their surgical treatment and the outcome differ considerably. Surgery is indicated for the cases resistant to medical treatment and for those suggestive of focal disease. Partial pancreatectomy can cure focal HI by resection of the adenomatous hyperplasia. Diffuse forms resistant to medical therapy require near-total pancreatectomy with high risk of postoperative diabetes mellitus and pancreatic insufficiency [20, 21].

The two histopathological forms correspond to two distinct molecular entities, implicating mainly the *SUR1* and *KIR6.2* genes. Different underlying genetic defects have been described previously [22, 25]. Focal HI is associated with a paternally inherited mutation in the ATP-sensitive potassium channel genes encoding the sulphonylurea receptor (ABCC8 or SUR1) or the inwardly rectifying potassium channel subunit (KCNJ11 or KIR6.2), both located in the 11p15.1 region, and loss of the maternal 11p15 allele restricted to the pancreatic lesion as well as a somatic reduction to homozygosity [15]. The diffuse form of HI is more heterogeneous and several genes are involved with autosomal recessive or, less frequently, dominant inheritance, namely *SUR1*, *Kir6.2* [14, 26, 27], glucokinase [28], glutamate dehydrogenase (with associated hyperammonaemia) [29], and most recently, short-chain L-3-hydroxyacyl-coenzyme A dehydrogenase [30]. Unfortunately, important clinical decisions regarding surgical treatment have to be taken before the results from mutational analyses are often available.

For several reasons, the distinction between the two forms of HI before surgery is difficult to perform: (a) contrary to adult pancreatic adenoma, focal lesions in infants are impossible to identify macroscopically by ultrasound, MRI or CT, as they are lobulated like the normal pancreatic parenchyma; (b) until recently, the localization of insulin hypersecretion before surgery was only possible through pancreatic venous catheterization to collect venous blood samples [pancreatic venous sampling (PVS)], latterly with additional intravenous stimulation of insulin secretion by calcium and tolbutamide to allow a pancreatic map of glucose, insulin and C peptide concentrations [31–35]. Even though PVS was relatively accurate (75%), the hyperglycaemic effect of general anaesthesia could prevent a satisfactory diagnostic evaluation. Also, PVS and pancreatic arterial calcium stimulation are invasive methods, technically difficult to perform, and requiring general anaesthesia. The concentrations of plasma glucose must be carefully maintained between 2 and 3 mmol/l before and during the PVS. Moreover, all medical treatments have to be stopped 5 days before this study. Using these methods, hypersecretion is considered diffuse when an increase in plasma insulin concentration is seen in more than one arterial territory and focal when this increase occurs in a single arterial territory. The area of hypersecretion is assumed to be in the territory supplied by the artery: gastroduodenal and superior mesenteric arteries for the pancreatic head, splenic artery for the pancreatic body and tail [33]. Due to the complexity of this approach, clinicians were keen to identify less invasive examinations to carry out differential diagnosis between focal and diffuse HI also allowing better localization of focal lesions to guide the surgeon.

L-Dihydroxyphenylalanine (L-DOPA) is a precursor of catecholamines which is converted to dopamine by the aromatic L-amino acid decarboxylase (AADC) enzyme. In addition to its role as a precursor of noradrenaline and adrenaline, dopamine is a transmitter substance in the central and peripheral nervous system. The capacity to take up and decarboxylate amine precursors such as L-DOPA or 5-hydroxytryptophan and store their biogenic amines (dopamine and serotonin) is characteristic of neuro-endocrine cells.

Pancreatic cells contain markers usually associated with neuro-endocrine cells, such as tyrosine hydroxylase, dopamine, neuronal dopamine transporter, vesicular dopamine transporter, monoamine oxidases A and B [36–38]. Pancreatic islets have been shown to take up L-DOPA and convert it to dopamine through AADC [39–41].

The term 'neuro-endocrine tumours' comprises a wide variety of rare tumour entities that may originate either from pure endocrine organs (e.g. pituitary adenomas), from pure nerve structures (e.g. neuroblastomas), or from elements of the diffuse (neuro)endocrine system such as all endocrine tumours of the gastro-entero-pancreatic tract. These neuro-endocrine disordered cells share similar cytochemical and ultrastructural characteristics. They have the capacity to take up dopamine precursors and convert them to amines or peptides, or both, which they store in secretory granules in the cytoplasm. Yet, it has been discovered that other cells throughout the body share this ability of amine precursor uptake and decarboxylation. The term 'amine precursor uptake and decarboxylation' has more lately been found to be inadequate, since several cell types included in the system do not metabolize amines. Furthermore, there is evidence that some amine precursor uptake and decarboxylation cell types are not of neural crest origin, but are derived from the endoderm [42]. So, HI, as all neuro-endocrine diseases, is able to take up amine precursors and to convert them into biogenic amines.

Positron emission tomography (PET) performed with [^{18}F]fluoro-L-DOPA has been extensively used to study the central dopaminergic system, mainly in Parkinson's disease. However, several recent studies have demonstrated the usefulness of this radiotracer to detect neuro-endocrine tumours such as phaeochromocytomas, thyroid medullary carcinomas or gastro-intestinal carcinoid tumours that usually contain secretory granules and have the ability to produce biogenic amines [42–46]. Based on the results of these studies, we assessed the use of [^{18}F]fluoro-L-DOPA PET in HI patients to detect the functional pancreatic islet tissue and evaluated the accuracy of this method to differentiate the 2 major histopathological forms of HI and replace PVS [47–49].

Materials and Methods

Patients

Fifty-four children (33 boys and 21 girls; age 1–24 months; median age 4.1 months) with HI were studied with [^{18}F]fluoro-L-DOPA PET. In all the cases, HI diagnosis was based upon persistent hypoglycaemia with low plasma ketone bodies and free fatty acids, together with measurable circulating insulin levels during hypoglycaemia episodes.

The patients fasted for at least 6 h prior to the PET study. Treatment with octreotide was stopped for at least 1 day and diazoxide for at least 2 days before the PET scan. In one case, the PET study was performed whilst receiving glucagon. During all PET studies, normoglycaemia was maintained through glucose infusion, which was carefully adjusted according to frequent blood glucose monitoring. Glucose infusion rates between 6.4 and 13.2 mg/kg/min were required. PET acquisition was performed under light sedation (pentobarbital with or without chloral).

Fifteen patients for whom [^{18}F]fluoro-L-DOPA uptake results strongly suggested focal HI and 9 patients with diffuse HI, resistant to medical treatment, had surgical resection. Pancreatic tissue obtained from resections was fixed in formalin, embedded in paraffin, and serial sections were studied by immunohistochemistry after a water bath antigen retrieval step [47, 48].

Data Acquisition

Magnetic Resonance Imaging

Thirty-one children underwent MRI of the abdomen using a 1.5-tesla imager (Sigma, GE, Healthcare, Milwaukee, Wisc., USA), and T_1-weighted spoiled gradient recalled acquisition in the steady state with inversion recovery was performed to allow 3-dimensional reconstruction of magnetic resonance images. MRI was used to reveal potential signal abnormalities in the pancreas and to allow coregistration between PET and MRI.

Positron Emission Tomography

The patients fasted for at least 6 h prior to the PET study and their medications were stopped for at least 72 h. During all PET studies, normoglycaemia was maintained by glucose infusion, which was carefully adjusted according to frequent blood glucose monitoring. Maximal glucose infusion rates between 6.4 and 13.2 mg/kg/min were needed. PET acquisition was performed under light sedation (pentobarbital with or without chloral).

The PET studies were performed using an ECAT EXACT HR+ scanner (Siemens Medical Solutions, Knoxville, Tenn., USA) which collects 63 simultaneous 2.4-mm-thick slices with an intrinsic in-plane resolution of 4.3 mm. The patients were placed in supine position in the scanner using a 3-dimensional laser alignment. To ensure the optimal position in the scanner and to avoid movement artefacts, the children should be comfortably immobilized during the PET acquisition by placing them in a vacuum mattress. The synthesis of [^{18}F]fluoro-L-DOPA followed a previously described electrophilic procedure [50]. Intravenous bolus injection of a mean of 4.0 MBq/kg [^{18}F]fluoro-L-DOPA was done 30–50 min before transmission acquisition.

Tissue attenuation was measured using three ^{68}Ge rod sources (approximately 450 MBq). Transmission scans (2-dimensional acquisition mode) lasted 2.5 min per bed position (field of view of 15 cm), with 2 or 3 steps, according to the height of the patient, from the neck to the hip. After segmentation, they were used for subsequent correction of attenuation of emission scans. Thorax-abdomen emission scans (3-dimensional acquisition mode) started between 45 and 65 min after the radiotracer injection; 2.5-min step acquisitions, 2 or 3 steps for 1 scan, were acquired over 30 min.

Data Analysis

The emission sets were corrected for scatter using a model-based correction, allowing simulation of the map of single scatter events. The images were reconstructed using an attenuation-weighted ordered-subset expectation maximization iterative algorithm with 4 iterations and 6 subsets. The final spatial resolution in reconstructed images was approximately 6.0 mm.

The reconstructed images were evaluated in a 3-dimensional display using axial, coronal, and sagittal views to visualize the pancreas, which invariably has a sufficient uptake of [^{18}F]fluoro-L-DOPA to distinguish it from the surrounding organs in the abdomen.

For each patient, all thorax-abdomen emission scans were assembled with bed position overlap and this integrated image was used to achieve the coregistration with MRI slices. Concerning MRI acquisitions, a specific field of view was determined to include the pancreas, the liver and the kidneys, which were the only organs visible in PET images in the abdominal area. A corresponding field of view was then extracted from PET images. Due to the low contrast observed between the kidneys and surrounding organs on MRI images, an enhancement of the grey-level intensity of these structures based on a manual segmentation of the kidneys was performed. Volume-based coregistration of PET and enhanced MRI images was done using mutual information as matching criterion [51–53]. Global rigid transformation was considered for the spatial alignment [54]. The coregistration task was evaluated visually using a fusion mode taking into account the superimposition of the liver and the kidneys in both modalities [55]. Finally, improvement of pancreatic uptake targeting was achieved by fusing anatomical MRI and functional co-aligned PET information on the pancreas.

Results

Pancreatic MRI studies were non-informative concerning the differentiation between focal and diffuse HI but confirmed the localization of the [^{18}F]fluoro-L-DOPA in the pancreas. PET images showed that most of the radioactivity accumulated in the kidneys and urinary bladder, the main elimination route of the radiotracer (fig. 1). Consequently, the high radioactivity in these organs, particularly in the left kidney, might increase the difficulty in identifying focal forms localized in the tail of the pancreas when the PET images alone are interpreted. Furthermore, in some patients, we observed a physiological radiotracer accumulation by the gall bladder and the biliary duct. The physiological accumulation was observed even if all patients fasted for at least 6 h before the PET examination and the image acquisition started between 45 and 60 min after the radiotracer injection. Coregistered MRI and PET images help localizing the hot spot with respect to the head, the body and the tail of the pancreas. However, one should account for possible coregistration errors between both modalities.

In 15 patients, a focal uptake of [^{18}F]fluoro-L-DOPA was observed in the pancreatic area (fig. 1a). In these patients, the area of the suspected pancreatic abnormality, based on imaging diagnosis, was biopsied. For 14 children, the frozen section confirmed that the histological abnormality was confined to the focal lesions, and a limited pancreatic resection was performed. The immunohistochemical analysis corroborated the PET data, showing that the distribution of abnormal β-cells was restricted to the adenomatous hyperplasia, in all but 1 patient. For 1 patient, no focal lesion was observed by the surgeon and the immunohistochemical analysis showed an atypical form of HI. For the 14 children with a focal lesion confirmed by immunohistochemical analysis, the limited pancreatic resection was followed by a clinical remission without carbohydrate intolerance.

For 39 children, a diffuse accumulation of [^{18}F]fluoro-L-DOPA (fig. 1b) was observed, and diffuse HI was suspected. Nine children were resistant to the medical

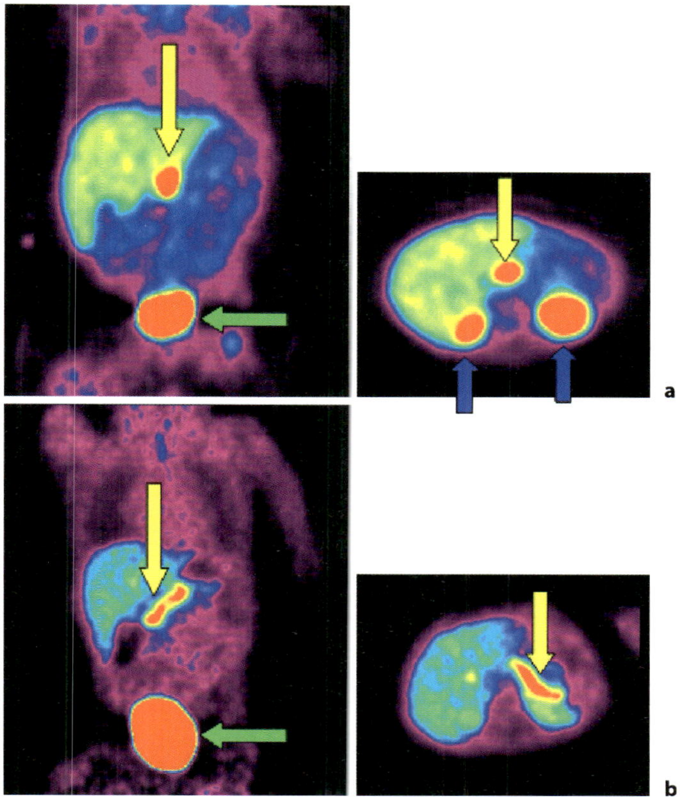

Fig. 1. a Patient with focal HI. A focal increased uptake of the radiotracer is visualized in the middle region of the pancreas on coronal and axial slices (yellow arrow). **b** A larger and diffuse uptake of the radiotracer is observed over the pancreatic area (yellow arrow). A physiological distribution of the radiotracer with a higher accumulation in the urinary bladder (green arrows) and kidneys (blue arrows) and a lower accumulation in the liver is also observed.

treatment and were submitted to surgery. In 7 cases, near-total pancreatectomy was performed and in 2 cases hemipancreatectomy, after frozen-section histological examination of multiple random pancreatic biopsies. The PET results were confirmed by histological data.

In 1 case, the PET study was performed under glucagon infusion and showed no uptake of the radiotracer in the pancreas.

Discussion

Our work shows that PET using [^{18}F]fluoro-L-DOPA positively differentiates focal from diffuse HI. When a focal uptake of [^{18}F]fluoro-L-DOPA was detected, the immunohistochemical data obtained on surgical resection confirmed the diagnosis of focal HI (14/15). On the other hand, when a diffuse pattern of [^{18}F]fluoro-L-DOPA was observed, the histological data from 7 of 9 operated children with diffuse HI exhibited a large distribution of the pathological β-cells throughout the pancreas. The histological findings corroborated the PET results in 93% of the focal forms and in

85% of the operated diffuse patients and illustrated a pancreas β-cell co-localization of pro-insulin and AADC in focal HI. Finally, 2 of the 3 atypical HI forms were identified by PET as diffuse HI and 1 as focal HI. Our results are consistent with those published recently by other groups. These authors estimated a 96% accuracy of [^{18}F]fluoro-L-DOPA PET in establishing the correct diagnosis of HI [56, 57].

In our work, the localization of the lesion was performed using PET images or fused PET and MRI images when available. MRI was not acquired using the same bed as for the PET study. As a consequence, the movements of the abdominal organs between the two imaging modalities are more pronounced than they would be if combined PET/CT was used for the acquisition of functional and anatomical images. However, MRI has the advantage of reducing the radiation dose exposure of the subject as compared to CT.

The 14 children with focal HI, who underwent limited pancreatectomy, showed normal postoperative blood glucose levels. At the present time, these 14 children are in clinical remission.

Seven children, with diffuse HI, had near-total pancreatectomy. Surgery was followed by a series of hypoglycaemic episodes with a variable degree of severity and frequency and almost all of these children developed diabetes mellitus.

The 3 operated, atypical HI forms presented a diffuse histological type pattern involving an area corresponding to half of the pancreas. However, sometimes hypoglycaemia is not cured by hemipancreatectomy. Nevertheless, hypoglycaemia can be medically controlled. One of the 3 cases identified as having the atypical form and submitted to hemipancreatectomy is currently in clinical remission whilst the other 2 children require continued treatment. The 30 children with a diffuse form of HI who were not operated on are maintained on a diet and medication.

The effect of the medications (octreotide and diazoxide) generally used for HI treatment on [^{18}F]fluoro-L-DOPA uptake was evaluated in 2 children: 1 with the diffuse form and 1 with the focal form. Both children had 2 PET studies: 1 on medication and 1 without medication. The uptake of [^{18}F]fluoro-L-DOPA remained unchanged between the 2 PET studies. Thus, in contrast to PVS, PET studies could be performed without stopping these medications. However, glucagon (a potent anti-hypoglycaemia agent) administration interferes with the uptake of [^{18}F]fluoro-L-DOPA: for 1 patient, this drug was not stopped before PET study and no pancreatic tracer uptake was observed. In a previous study, we had investigated the relationship between insulin and AADC localization in normal human pancreas at several ages or stages of development and in tissue from focal and diffuse HI lesions [48]. A strong correlation between the co-localization of these 2 parameters was observed for focal forms. This correlation is associated with the close anatomical relationship between pancreatic α- and β-cells, and might explain the absence of [^{18}F]fluoro-L-DOPA uptake under glucagon perfusion. In fact, the interaction between insulin and glucagon release within the islet of Langerhans is well known [58]. Glucagon, interfering with β-cell activity, will probably also interfere with AADC activity [59, 60].

In conclusion, [^{18}F]fluoro-L-DOPA PET has become the preferred method for the differentiation between focal and diffuse HI. In contradistinction to PVS, PET is non-invasive and atraumatic. Furthermore, PET studies can be performed without stopping medication (except for glucagon) and under light sedation. PET results were concordant with the immunohistochemical analysis performed after partial (focal HI) or near-total pancreatectomy (diffuse HI resistant to medical treatment) for 21 of 24 children submitted to surgery.

Acknowledgements

We are greatly indebted to the chemical and nursing staff of Service Hospitalier Frédéric Joliot, Orsay, France. We are particularly grateful to the GIS-Institut des Maladies Rares (Paris) and the Fondation Lejeune.

References

1 Rahier J, Falt K, Muntefering H, Becker K, Gepts W, Falkmer S: The basic structural lesion of persistent neonatal hypoglycemia with hyperinsulinism: deficiency of pancreatic D cells or hyperactivity of B cells? Diabetologia 1984;26:282–289.

2 Goossens A, Gepts W, Saudubray JM, Bonnefont JP, Nihoul-Fekete, Heitz PU, Kloppel G: Diffuse and focal nesidioblastosis. A clinicopathological study of 24 patients with persistent neonatal hyperinsulinemic hypoglycemia. Am J Surg Pathol 1989;13: 766–775.

3 Sempoux C, Guiot Y, Lefevre A, Nihoul-Fékété C, Jaubert F, Saudubray JM, Rahier J: Neonatal hyperinsulinemic hypoglycemia: heterogeneity of the syndrome and keys for differential diagnosis. J Clin Endocrinol Metab 1988;83:1455–1461.

4 Menni F, De Lonlay P, Sevin C, Touati G, Peigne C, Barbier V, Nihoul-Fekete C, Saudubray JM, Robert JJ: Neurologic outcomes of 90 neonates and infants with persistent hyperinsulinemic hypoglycemia. Pediatrics 2001;107:476–479.

5 De Lonlay-Debeney P, Poggi-Travert F, Fournet JC, Sempoux C, Vici CD, Brunelle F, Touati G, Rahier J, Junien C, Nihoul-Fekete C, Robert JJ, Saudubray JM: Clinical features of 52 neonates with hyperinsulinism. N Engl J Med 1999;340:1169–1175.

6 Stanley CA: Hyperinsulinism in infants and children. Pediatr Clin North Am 1997;44:363–374.

7 Aynsley-Green A, Polak JM, Bloom SR, Gough MH, Keeling J, Ashcroft SJ, Turner RC, Baum JD: Nesidioblastosis of the pancreas: definition of the syndrome and the management of the severe neonatal hyperinsulinaemic hypoglycaemia. Arch Dis Child 1981;56:496–508.

8 Finegold DN, Stanley CA, Baker L: Glycemic response to glucagon during fasting hypoglycemia: an aid in the diagnosis of hyperinsulinism. J Pediatr 1980;96:257–259.

9 Hirsch HJ, Loo S, Evans N, Crigler JF, Filler RM, Gabbay KH: Hypoglycemia of infancy and nesidioblastosis. Studies with somatostatin. N Engl J Med 1977;296:1323–1326.

10 Glaser B, Hirsch HJ, Landau H: Persistent hyperinsulinemic hypoglycemia of infancy: long-term octreotide treatment without pancreatectomy. J Pediatr 1993;123:644–650.

11 Thornton PS, Alter CA, Katz LE, Baker L, Stanley CA: Short- and long-term use of octreotide in the treatment of congenital hyperinsulinism. J Pediatr 1993;123:637–643.

12 De Lonlay P, Fournet JC, Touati G, Groos MS, Martin D, Sevin C, Delagne V, Mayaud C, Chigot V, Sempoux C, Brusset MC, Laborde K, Bellane-Chantelot C, Vassault A, Rahier J, Junien C, Brunelle F, Nihoul-Fekete C, Saudubray JM, Robert JJ: Heterogeneity of persistent hyperinsulinaemic hypoglycaemia. A series of 175 cases. Eur J Pediatr 2002; 161:37–48.

13 Thomas PM, Cote GJ, Wohllk N, Haddad B, Mathew PM, Rabl W, Aguilar-Bryan L, Gagel RF, Bryan J: Mutations in the sulfonylurea receptor gene in familial persistent hyperinsulinemic hypoglycemia of infancy. Science 1995;268:426–429.

14 Nestorowicz A, Wilson BA, Schoor KP, Inoue H, Glaser B, Landau H, et al: Mutations in the sulfonylurea receptor gene are associated with familial hyperinsulinism in Ashkenazi Jews. Hum Mol Genet 1996;5:1813–1822.

15 De Lonlay P, Fournet JC, Rahier J, Gross-Morand MS, Poggi-Travert F, Foussier V, Bonnefont JP, Brusset MC, Brunelle F, Robert JJ, Nihoul-Fekete C, Saudubray JM, Junien C: Somatic deletion of the imprinted 11p15 region in sporadic persistent hyperinsulinemic hypoglycemia of infancy is specific of focal adenomatous hyperplasia and endorses partial pancreatectomy. J Clin Invest 1997;100:802–807.

16 Verkarre V, Fournet JC, De Lonlay P, Gross-Morand MS, Devillers M, Rahier J, Brunelle F, Robert JJ, Nihoul-Fekete C, Saudubray JM, Junien C: Paternal mutation of the sulfonylurea receptor (SUR1) gene and maternal loss of 11p15 imprinted genes lead to persistent hyperinsulinism in focal adenomatous hyperplasia. J Clin Invest 1998;102:1286–1291.

17 Fournet JC, Mayaud C, De Lonlay P, Gross-Morand MS, Verkarre V, Castanet M, Devillers M, Rahier J, Brunelle F, Robert JJ, Nihoul-Fekete C, Saudubray JM, Junien C: Unbalanced expression of 11p15 imprinted genes in focal forms of congenital hyperinsulinism: association with a reduction to homozygosity of a mutation in ABCC8 or KCNJ11. Am J Pathol 2001;158:2177–2184.

18 De Lonlay P, Simon A, Galmiche-Rolland L, Giurgea I, Verkarre V, Aigrain Y, Santiago-Ribeiro MJ, Polak M, Robert JJ, Bellanne-Chantelot, Brunelle F, Nihoul-Fekete C, Jaubert F: Neonatal hyperinsulinism: clinicopathologic correlation. Hum Pathol 2007;38:387–399.

19 De Lonlay P, Benelli C, Fouque F, Ganguly A, Aral B, Dionisi-Vici C, Touati G, Heinrichs C, Rabier D, Kamoun P, Robert JJ, Stanley C, Saudubray JM: Hyperinsulinism and hyperammonemia syndrome: report of twelve unrelated patients. Pediatr Res 2001;50:353–357.

20 Filler RM, Weinberg MJ, Cutz E, Wesson DE, Ehrlich RM: Current status of pancreatectomy for persistent idiopathic neonatal hypoglycemia due to islet cell dysplasia. Prog Pediatr Surg 1991;26:60–75.

21 Fékété CN, De Lonlay P, Jaubert F, Rahier J, Brunelle F, Saudubray: The surgical management of congenital hyperinsulinemic hypoglycemia in infancy. J Pediatr Surg 2004;39:267–269.

22 Thornton PS, MacMullen C, Ganguly A, Ruchelli E, Steinkrauss L, Crane A, Aguilar-Bryan L, Stanley CA: Clinical and molecular characterization of a dominant form of congenital hyperinsulinism caused by a mutation in the high-affinity sulfonylurea receptor. Diabetes 2003;52:2403–2410.

23 Glaser B, Ryan F, Donath M, Landau H, Stanley CA, Baker L, Barton, Thornton PS: Hyperinsulinism caused by paternal-specific inheritance of a recessive mutation in the sulfonylurea-receptor gene. Diabetes 1999;48:1652–1657.

24 Sempoux C, Guiot Y, Dahan K, Moulin P, Stevens M, Lambot V, de Lonlay P, Fournet JC, Junien C, Jaubert F, Nihoul-Fekete C, Saudubray JM, Rahier J: The focal form of persistent hyperinsulinemic hypoglycemia of infancy: morphological and molecular studies show structural and functional differences with insulinoma. Diabetes 2003;52:784–794.

25 De Lonlay P, Giurgea I, Sempoux C, Touati G, Jaubert F, Rahier J, Ribeiro M, Brunelle F, Nihoul-Fekete C, Robert JJ, Saudubray JM, Stanley C, Bellanne-Chantelot C: Dominantly inherited hyperinsulinaemic hypoglycaemia. J Inherit Metab Dis 2005;28:267–276.

26 Thomas PM, Cote GJ, Wohllk N, Mathew PM, Gagel RF: The molecular basis for familial persistent hyperinsulinemic hypoglycemia of infancy. Proc Assoc Am Physicians 1996;108:14–19.

27 Huopio H, Reimann F, Ashfield R, Komulainen J, Lenko HL, Rahier J, Vauhkonen I, Kere J, Laakso M, Ashcroft F, Otonkoski T: Dominantly inherited hyperinsulinism caused by a mutation in the sulfonylurea receptor type 1. J Clin Invest 2000;106:897–906.

28 Glaser B, Kesaven P, Heyman M, Davis E, Cuesta A, Buchs A, Stanley CA, Thornton PS, Permutt MA, Matschinsky FM, Herold KC: Familial hyperinsulinism caused by an activating glucokinase mutation. N Engl J Med 1998;338:226–230.

29 Stanley CA, Lieu YK, Hsu BY, Burlina AB, Greenberg CR, Hopwood NJ, Perlman K, Rich BH, Zammarchi E, Poncz M: Hyperinsulinism and hyperammonemia in infants with regulatory mutations of the glutamate dehydrogenase gene. N Engl J Med 1998;338:1352–1357.

30 Clayton PT, Eaton S, Aynsley-Green A, Edginton M, Hussain K, Krywawych S, Datta V, Malingre HE, Berger R, van den Berg IE: Hyperinsulinism in short-chain L-3-hydroxyacyl-CoA dehydrogenase deficiency reveals the importance of beta-oxidation in insulin secretion. J Clin Invest 2001;108:457–465.

31 Brunelle F, Negre V, Barth MO, Fekete CN, Czernichow P, Saudubray JM, Kuntz F, Tach T, Lallemand D: Pancreatic venous samplings in infants and children with primary hyperinsulinism. Pediatr Radiol 1989;19:100–103.

32 Dubois J, Brunelle F, Touati G, Sebag G, Nuttin C, Thach T, Nihoul-Fekete C, Rahier J, Saudubray JM: Hyperinsulinism in children: diagnostic value of pancreatic venous sampling correlated with clinical, pathological and surgical outcome in 25 cases. Pediatr Radiol 1995;25:512–516.

33 Chigot V, De Lonlay P, Nassogne MC, Laborde K, Delagne V, Fournet JC, Nihoul-Fékété C, Saudubray JM, Brunelel F: Pancreatic arterial calcium stimulation in the diagnosis and localisation of persistent hyperinsulinemic hypoglycaemia of infancy. Pediatr Radiol 2001;31:650–655.

34 Giurgea I, Laborde K, Touati G, Bellanne-Chantelot C, Nassogne MC, Sempoux C, Jaubert F, Khoa N, Chigot V, Rahier J, Brunelle F, Nihoul-Fékété C, Dunne MJ, Stanley C, Saudubray JM, Robert JJ, de Lonlay P: Acute insulin responses to calcium and tolbutamide do not differentiate focal from diffuse congenital hyperinsulinism. J Clin Endocrinol Metab 2004;89:925–929.

35 Stanley CA, Thornton PS, Ganguly A, MacMullen C, Underwood P, Bhatia P, Steinkrauss L, Wanner L, Kaye R, Ruchelli E, Suchi M, Adzick NS: Preoperative evaluation of infants with focal or diffuse congenital hyperinsulinism by intravenous acute insulin response tests and selective pancreatic arterial calcium stimulation. J Clin Endocrinol Metab 2004;89:288–296.

36 Lemmer K, Ahnert-Hilger G, Hopfner M, et al: Expression of dopamine receptors and transporter in neuroendocrine gastrointestinal tumor cells. Life Sci 2002;71:667–678.

37 Rodriguez MJ, Saura J, Finch CC, Mahy N, Billet EE: Localization of monoamine oxidase A and B in human pancreas, thyroid and adrenal glands. J Histochem Cytochem 2000;48:147–151.

38 Orlefors H, Sundin A, Fasth KJ, Oberg K, Langstrom B, Eriksson B, Bergstrom M: Demonstration of high monoaminoxidase-A levels in neuroendocrine gastroenteropancreatic tumors in vitro and in vivo-tumor visualization using positron emission tomography with ^{11}C-harmine. Nucl Med Biol 2003;30:669–679.

39 Oei HK, Gazdar AF, Minna JD, Weir GC, Baylin SB: Clonal analysis of insulin and somatostatin secretion and L-dopa decarboxylase expression by a rat islet cell tumor. Endocrinology 1983;112:1070–1075.

40 Lindstrom P: Aromatic-L-amino-acid decarboxylase activity in mouse pancreatic islets. Biochim Biophys Acta 1986;884:276–281.

41 Borelli MI, Villar MJ, Orezzoli A, Gagliardino JJ: Presence of DOPA decarboxylase and its localisation in adult rat pancreatic islet cells. Diabetes Metab 1997;23:161–163.

42 Oei HK, De Jong M, Krenning EP: Gastroenteropancreatic neuroendocrine tumors; in Feinendegen LE, Shreeve WW, Eckelman WC, Bahk YW, Wagner HN (eds): Molecular Nuclear Medicine. Heidelberg, Springer, 2003, pp 385–397.

43 Hoegerle S, Altehoefer C, Ghanem N, Brink I, Moser E, Nitzsche E: ^{18}F-DOPA positron emission tomography for tumour detection in patients with medullary thyroid carcinoma and elevated calcitonin levels. Eur J Nucl Med 2001;28:64–71.

44 Hoegerle S, Altehoefer C, Ghanem N, et al: Whole-body ^{18}F DOPA PET for detection of gastrointestinal carcinoid tumors. Radiology 2001;220:373–380.

45 Hoegerle S, Nitzsche E, Altehoefer C, et al: Pheochromocytomas detection with ^{18}F DOPA whole-body PET – initial results. Radiology 2002;222:507–512.

46 Hoegerle S, Ghanem N, Altehoefer C, Schipper J, Brink I, Moser E, Neumann HP: ^{18}F-DOPA positron emission tomography for the detection of glomus tumours. Eur J Nucl Med Mol Imaging 2003;30:689–694.

47 Ribeiro MJ, De Lonlay P, Delzescaux T, Boddaert N, Jaubert F, Bourgeois S, Dollé F, Nihoul-Fékété C, Syrota A, Brunelle F: Characterization of hyperinsulinism in infancy assessed with PET and ^{18}F-fluoro-L-DOPA. J Nucl Med 2005;46:560–566.

48 De Lonlay P, Simon-Carre A, Ribeiro MJ, Boddaert N, Giurgea I, Laborde K, Bellanne-Chantelot C, Verkarre V, Polak M, Rahier J, Syrota A, Seidenwurm D, Nihoul-Fekete C, Robert JJ, Brunelle F, Jaubert F: Congenital hyperinsulinism: pancreatic [^{18}F]fluoro-L-DOPA positron emission tomography and immunohistochemistry study of DOPA decarboxylase and insulin secretion. J Clin Endocrinol Metab 2006;291:933–940.

49 Ribeiro MJ, Boddaert N, Bellanné-Chantelot C, Bourgeois S, Valayannopoulos V, Delzescaux T, Jaubert F, Nihoul-Fékété C, Brunelle F, De Lonlay P: The added value of [^{18}F]fluoro-L-DOPA PET in the diagnosis of hyperinsulinism of infancy: a retrospective study involving 49 children. Eur J Nucl Med Mol Imaging, in press.

50 Dollé F, Demphel S, Hinnen F, Fournier D, Vaufrey F, Crouzel C: 6-[^{18}F]Fluoro-L-DOPA by radiofluorodestannylation: a short and simple synthesis of a new labelling precursor. J Labelled Comp Radiopharm 1998;XLI:105–114.

51 Wells WM, Viola PV, Atsumi H, Nakajima S, Kikinis R: Multi-modal volume registration by maximization of mutual information. Med Image Anal 1996;1:35–51.

52 Maes F, Collignon A, Vandermeulen D, Marechal G, Suetens R: Multimodality image registration by maximization of mutual information. IEEE Trans Med Imaging 1997;16:187–198.

53 Pluim JPW, Maintz JBA, Viergever MA: Mutual-information-based registration of medical images: a survey. IEEE Trans Med Imaging 2003;22:986–1004.

54 Maintz J, Viergever M: A survey for medical image registration. Med Image Anal 1998;2:1–36.
55 Lemke AJ, Niehues SM, Hosten N, Amthauer H, Boehmig M, Stroszczynski C, Rohlfing T, Rosewicz S, Felix R: Retrospective digital image fusion of multidetector CT and ^{18}F-FDG PET/clinical value in pancreatic lesions – A prospective study with 104 patients. J Nucl Med 2004;45:1279–1286.
56 Hardy OT, Hernandez-Pampaloni M, Saffer JR, Suchi M, Ruchelli E, Zhuang H, Ganguly A, Freifelder R, Adzick NS, Alavi A, Stanley CA: Diagnosis and localization of focal congenital hyperinsulinism by ^{18}F-fluodopa PET scan. J Pediatr 2007;150:140–145.
57 Otonkoski T, Nanto-Salonen K, Seppanen M, Veijola R, Huopio H, Hussain K, Tapanainen P, Eskola O, Parkkola R, Ekstrom K, Guiot Y, Rahier J, Laakso M, Rintala R, Nuutila P, Minn H: Noninvasive diagnosis of focal hyperinsulinism of infancy with [^{18}F]-DOPA positron emission tomography. Diabetes 2006;55:13–18.
58 Asplin CM, Paquette TL, Palmer JP: In vivo inhibition of glucagon secretion by paracrine beta cell activity in man. J Clin Invest 1981;68:314–318.
59 Moens K, Berger V, Ahn JM, Van Schravendijk C, Hruby VJ, Pipeleers D, Schuit F: Assessment of the role of interstitial glucagon in the acute glucose secretory responsiveness of in situ pancreatic beta-cells. Diabetes 2002;51:669–675.
60 Hussain K, Bryan J, Christesen HT, Brusgaard K, Aguilar-Bryan L: Serum glucagon counterregulatory hormonal response to hypoglycemia is blunted in congenital hyperinsulinism. Diabetes 2005;54: 2946–2951.

Dr. Maria-João Ribeiro
Frédéric Joliot Hospital, Biomedical Imaging Institute
Life Sciences Division, CEA, 4, place du Général Leclerc
FR–91406 Orsay (France)
Tel. +33 1 69 86 78 00, Fax +33 1 69 86 77 28, E-Mail maria-joao.ribeiro@cea.fr

Shield JPH, Scharfmann R (eds): Development of the Pancreas and Neonatal Diabetes.
Endocr Dev. Basel, Karger, 2007, vol 12, pp 67–74

Insulin Pump Therapy in Neonatal Diabetes

Nadia Tubiana-Rufi

Department of Endocrinology and Diabetology, Robert Debré Hospital, AP-HP, Paris, France

Abstract

Neonatal diabetes mellitus is rare. Typically, infants are of low birth weight and develop hyperglycemia requiring exogenous insulin within the first 6 weeks. Although pediatricians face numerous difficulties in managing insulin therapy at this age, very few data are available on possible methods of insulin delivery in neonatal diabetes. We report our experience over 18 years of continuous subcutaneous insulin infusion (CSII) in cases of neonatal diabetes requiring insulin therapy for more than 15 days (n = 17; 8 permanent). CSII therapy in neonatal diabetes allows easy adaptation of insulin delivery, closely following the current feeding regimen (a basal infusion only being needed when using continuous enteral or parenteral feeding; preprandial boluses being started with intermittent bottle feeding). Management of the very small insulin doses (for example: bolus = 0.20 U and basal rate = 0.02 U/h) required is possible after insulin dilution (5–10 U/ml) and is more accurate with CSII than with syringes. Controlling blood glucose with few hypoglycemic events, which are particularly frequent and dangerous at this age, is more efficient with CSII than with injections. Infants tolerate the subcutaneous infusion lines well and we did not observe any side effects. For all children, CSII was utilized throughout the whole period of insulin therapy. In conclusion, during the neonatal period, and under the supervision of an experienced team, CSII is safe, more physiological and accurate and easier to manage than injections allowing easier matching of the insulin requirements of a newborn.

Neonatal diabetes mellitus is extremely rare (1/400,000 births in Europe) [1]. Typically, infants are of low birth weight and develop hyperglycemia requiring exogenous insulin within the first 6 postnatal weeks [2]. Although pediatricians face several difficulties in managing insulin therapy at this age, few data are available on the mode of insulin delivery in this condition [3, 4].

Eighteen years ago, in our center at Robert Debré Hospital, under the direction of Prof. Paul Czernichow, we developed the technique of continuous subcutaneous insulin infusion (CSII) in pediatric patients, especially in young children, demonstrating the feasibility of pump therapy while abrogating severe hypoglycemia in this age group [5, 6]. These positive experiences in young children led us to initiate pump therapy in neonates in whom diabetes is particularly difficult to manage with insulin injections [7].

We report the lessons drawn from our experience of CSII in the cases of neonatal diabetes requiring subcutaneous insulin therapy for more than 15 days. During the last 18 years we have initiated CSII in 17 newborns: 8 were transient and 9 permanent cases of neonatal diabetes. All patients were negative for type 1 diabetes-related autoantibodies. Results of molecular genetic studies [8–11] were available in 16 patients. Mutations were identified on chromosome 6 in 3 children, in Kir6.2 in 4 children, in SUR1 in 3, and not found in 6 cases (including 2 patients with IPF1-negative pancreas agenesis). All patients had pump therapy throughout the entire period of insulin treatment: in the 8 transient neonatal diabetes cases, insulin was required for 2 months to 1.7 years, and in the permanent cases for 3 months (in the most recent case) up to 13 years of follow-up.

Specific Challenges of Insulin Therapy in Neonatal Diabetes

Insulin therapy in neonatal diabetes is challenging due to:
- the need for extremely low doses of insulin per day, relative to the weight of neonates, and the peculiar very low basal rate requirements, especially during the night;
- the fact that prandial insulin administration has to be tailored to frequent and high-carbohydrate content meals, which vary in number through the first postnatal weeks (from 8 to 4 meals per day);
- the increased tendency to hypoglycemia in infants, which can be frequent and particularly dangerous for brain development;
- the need for these infants, often born small for gestational age, to attain sufficient weight gain which requires a high caloric intake and sufficient insulinization to allow catch-up growth.

Management of Continuous Subcutaneous Insulin Infusion in Neonatal Diabetes

Patients and Methods

Clinical characteristics are provided for a selection of 11 cases of neonatal diabetes in table 1, showing frequent intrauterine growth retardation, metabolic status at diagnosis (ketoacidosis in 3 cases), and ages at diabetes diagnosis and at initiation of CSII.

Table 1. Characteristics of the patients

Case No.	Sex	Birth weight, g; term, weeks	Metabolic status before insulin therapy	Age at insulin therapy, days	Age at initiation of CSII, days
1	F	2,530; 38	BG = 19 mmol/l ketonuria = 0	2 (i.v.)	7
2	F	1,430; 38	BG = 34 mmol/l ketonuria = 0	15 (i.v.)	17
3	M	1,200; 33	BG = 13 mmol/l ketonuria = 0	21 (s.c. inj. ×4/day)	26
4	F	2,100; 38	BG = 30 mmol/l ketonuria = 0	42 (i.v./s.c. inj. ×2/day)	55
5	M	3,040; 40	BG = 44.5 mmol/l ketonuria = 0	32 (i.v.)	33
6	F	1,890; 37.5	BG = 32 mmol/l ketonuria = 0	11 (i.v.)	13
7	F	1,200; 35	BG = 20 mmol/l ketonuria = 0	1 (i.v.)	34
8	M	1,600; 35.5	BG = 23 mmol/l ketonuria = 0	2 (i.v.)	24
9	M	3,150; 38.5	BG = 64 mmol/l ketoacidosis	38 (i.v.)	43
10	M	3,030; 41	BG = 21 mmol/l ketoacidosis	52 (i.v.)	56
11	M	2,590; 39.5	BG = 52 mmol/l ketoacidosis	120 (i.v.)	125

Cases 3, 4, 7, 8 were referred to our department several days after subcutaneous insulin injection therapy, which failed to control blood glucose (BG) levels (hypo/hyperglycemia).

Pump therapy was initiated a few days after intravenous insulin infusion, except in 4 cases who were referred to our department after failure to control blood glucose (BG) levels with subcutaneous injection therapy.

Practical aspects of insulin therapy management are described in what follows. During the first few days, the daily insulin dose requirement was evaluated with intravenous insulin and glucose infusions. When good glycemic control was obtained, CSII therapy was started. Different types of pumps were used, mainly Minimed 507, 508, and 512 (Medtronic Mininimed, Boulogne, France). Due to the low insulin requirements in these babies, the soluble or short-acting analogue insulin was diluted (5–10 IU/ml). Infusion sites were thighs or arms or the upper part of the back, and several types of infusion sets were used over the years (more recently: Quickset® and Silhouette®, Medtronic Minimed).

Table 2. Insulin doses during the first month of CSII

Case No.	Total daily dose, U/kg/day		
	T0 CSII	after 15 days	after 1 month
1	0.57 (100)[1]	0.96 (100)[1]	0.45 (100)[1]
2	0.70 (100)[1]	0.29 (100)[1]	0.40 (36)
3	0.37 (100)[1]	0.90 (100)[1]	0.60 (30)
4	0.73 (42)	1.0 (40)	0.65 (35)
5	0.40 (100)[1]	0.36 (32)	0.35 (31.5)
6	1.0 (100)[1]	0.6 (50)	0.8 (40)
7	0.6 (100)[1]	0.55 (100)[1]	0.47 (40)
8	0.42 (50)	0.54 (50)	0.25 (40)
9	0.48 (30)	0.76 (30)	0.66 (30)
10	1.0 (23)	1.2 (22)	1.1 (20)
11	0.48 (27)	1.4 (22.5)	1.06 (28)

Figures in parentheses indicate the daily basal rate (percent of total daily dose).
[1] Under enteral continuous feeding.

Results

Insulin Strategy

Insulin strategy for starting on CSII depends on the feeding conditions (tables 1 and 2):

- under enteral continuous feeding, the basal infusion accounts for 100% of the total daily dose (monitoring of BG every 3–4 h);
- when bottle feeding, the basal rate accounts for around 30% of the total daily dose (table 2, mean at 1 month in 10 patients = 33%) and the boluses for 70% of the total daily dose, with the same dose given before each meal (8, then 7, then 6 and 5 meals); BG is monitored before each meal and at 3 or 4 a.m.; the basal rate is thereafter adjusted to the night BG measurements and boluses are adjusted to postprandial BG measurements.

The total daily dose is established according to BG measurements, sufficient weight gain and is adjusted to the evolution of the number and content of the meals. We found that it could vary widely from 0.29 to 1.4 U/kg/day (table 2).

Blood Glucose Control

Estimates of long-term glycemic control cannot be based on HbA_{1c} levels, due to the high content of fetal hemoglobin during the first months of life.

BG control was assessed during the first month of CSII therapy in 5 patients. Using an average of 241 BG measurements per month, the mean BG level per month was 173 mg/dl (9.6 mmol/l), the mean number of hypoglycemic events (<60 mg/dl,

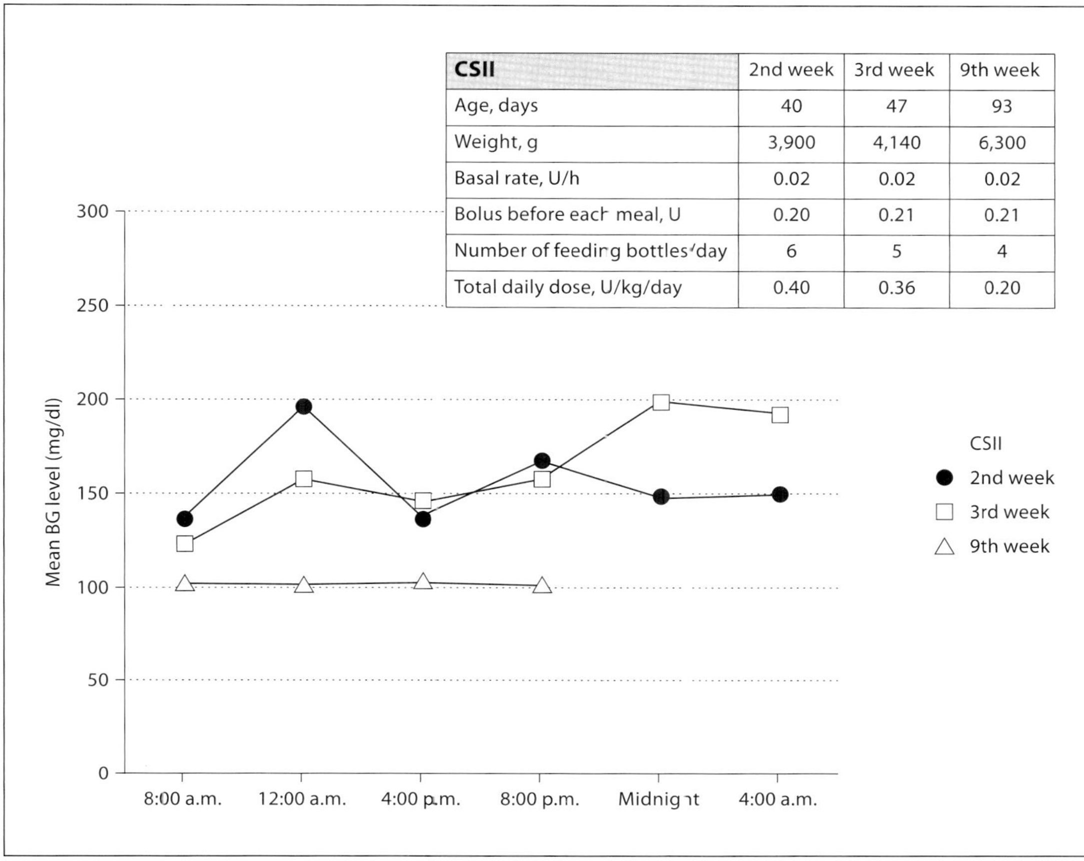

CSII	2nd week	3rd week	9th week
Age, days	40	47	93
Weight, g	3,900	4,140	6,300
Basal rate, U/h	0.02	0.02	0.02
Bolus before each meal, U	0.20	0.21	0.21
Number of feeding bottles/day	6	5	4
Total daily dose, U/kg/day	0.40	0.36	0.20

Fig. 1. Mean weekly BG profiles, weight and insulin doses during the 2nd and 3rd week (hospital) and 9th week (home) of CSII (case No. 5).

3.3 mmol/l) per month was 4.2 (1.6%), and no severe hypoglycemic events or episodes of ketoacidosis occurred. Details are given for case number 5 in figures 1 and 2 illustrating the progressive improvement of glucose control without hypoglycemia, the good weight gain and the low basal and bolus doses required.

Tolerance

Tolerance of the infusion sites was good and we did not observe any side effects.

For all children, CSII was utilized throughout the whole period of insulin therapy. No episodes of severe hypoglycemia or ketoacidosis were observed during the whole period of pump therapy after initial and continuous education from our experienced team.

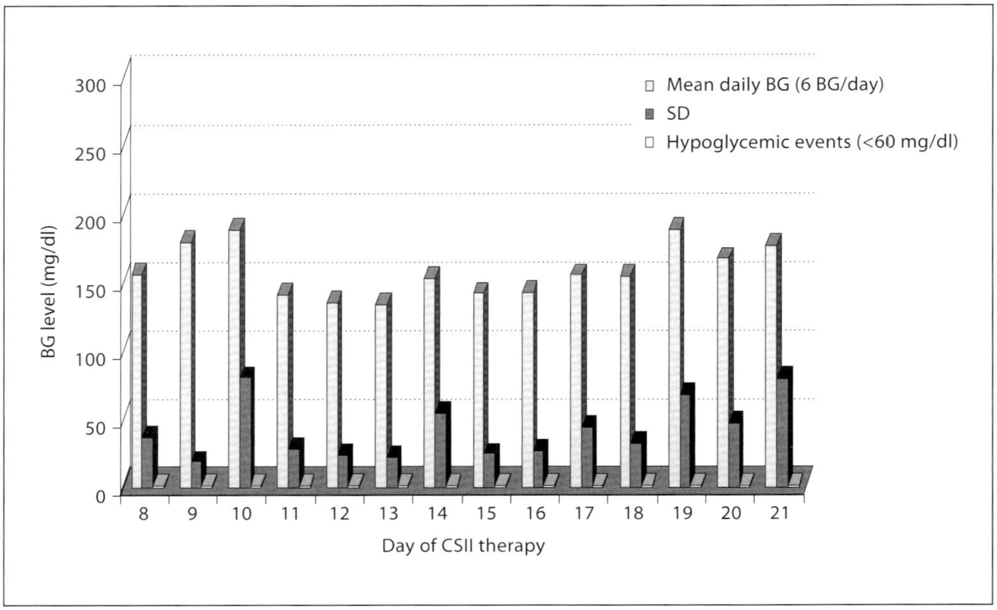

Fig. 2. Mean daily BG and hypoglycemia frequency during the 2nd and 3rd week (in hospital) of CSII therapy (case No. 5).

Discussion

The use of CSII therapy in neonatal diabetes gives great flexibility in providing dosage requirements effectively both for continuous enteral or parenteral feeding and for intermittent bottle feeding.

Management of very small insulin doses is possible after dilution (5–10 U/ml) and is more accurate with CSII than with syringes or pens. Achieving good glycemic control with few hypoglycemia episodes, which are particularly frequent and dangerous at this age, is more efficient with CSII than with injections (4 of our cases had previously failed intermittent, subcutaneous therapy). The infants tolerated CSII well and no complications occurred. CSII is more comfortable for babies, which is appreciated by the parents. Catheters are inserted every 2–3 days instead of 2 or more injections per day with syringes or pens.

Technical difficulties can be encountered, due to the lack of subcutaneous tissue in babies, especially in those born small for gestational age, all the more since available needles for inserting infusion sets are too long for babies. However, catheters without needles are well tolerated and more comfortable than metallic needles. Catheter insertion sites and infusion sets must be chosen according to the subcutaneous thickness. Long flexible Teflon catheters (Silhouette®, Medtronic Minimed) are more suitable for babies with little subcutaneous tissue, allowing good stability and longevity (3 days). The use of topical local anesthetic for catheter insertion is recommended to allay parental concerns.

The main difficulties we encountered were not related to the CSII therapy but to the psychological impact of the diagnosis on parents who are often shocked by the underlying diagnosis and worried about the long-term prognosis. We have utilized specific psychological support in this context. Frequent BG monitoring is required as babies often lack the classical symptoms of hypoglycemia.

Treatment success depends on adequate education and supervision of care given. A specialized multidisciplinary pediatric diabetes team including a pediatrician, dietician, nurse educator, psychologist and social worker is needed to give adequate and continuing counseling and education to parents and caregivers of very young children. Frequent contact between the family and the pediatric team is the key to achieving good metabolic control without acute complications. A 24-hour telephone hotline helps minimize acute metabolic complications or hospitalizations.

Conclusions

During the neonatal period, CSII therapy is safe, more physiological and accurate and easier to manage than intermittent injections. It succeeds in controlling BG with few hypoglycemic episodes, which are particularly frequent and dangerous at this age.

CSII therapy in neonatal diabetes needs to be managed or supervised by an experienced pediatric team of physicians and nurses used to dealing with diabetes in infancy and pump therapy in children.

Acknowledgements

Insulin pump therapy in the cases of neonatal diabetes was conducted in the Department of Endocrinology and Diabetology at Robert Debré Hospital, Paris, France, directed by Prof. Paul Czernichow from 1988 to 2006. We thank all pediatricians participating in the care of neonatal diabetes: Prof. Michel Polak, Drs. Geraldine Munz-Licha, Nadine Lucidarme, Marie-Aline Guitteny, Mireille Castanet, Sophie Guilmin Crepon, Isabelle Legac and the nursing team of the Department of Endocrinology at Robert Debré Hospital, Paris, especially Mrs. Laurence Leridon. Molecular genetic studies were performed by Helene Cave (Department of Genetics, Robert Debré Hospital, Paris) and Martine Vaxillaire (Institut Pasteur, Lille).

References

1 Von Mühlendahl KE, Herkenhoff H: Long-term course of neonatal diabetes. N Engl J Med 1995;333: 704–708.

2 Metz C, Cave H, Bertrand AM, Deffert C, Gueguen-Giroux B, Czernichow P, Polak M; NDM French Study Group, Neonatal diabetes mellitus: Neonatal diabetes mellitus: chromosomal analysis in transient and permanent cases. J Pediatr 2002; 141:483–489.

3 Mitamura R, Kimura H, Murakami Y, Nagaya K, Makita Y, Okuno A: Ultralente insulin treatment of transient neonatal diabetes mellitus. J Pediatr 1996; 128:268–270.

4 Olinder AL, Kernell A, Smide B: Treatment with CSII in two infants with neonatal diabetes mellitus. Pediatr Diabetes 2006;7:284–288.

5 Tubiana-Rufi N, de Lonlay P, Bloch J, Czernichow P: Remission of severe hypoglycemia incidents in young diabetic children treated with subcutaneous infusion. Arch Pediatr 1996;3:969–976.

6 Tubiana-Rufi N, Coutant R, Bloch J, Munz-Licha G, Delcroix C, Limal JM, Czernichow P: Special management of insulin lispro in continuous subcutaneous insulin infusion in young diabetic children: a randomized cross-over study. Horm Res 2004;62: 265–271.

7 Tubiana-Rufi N, Munz-Licha G, Polak M, Czernichow P: Continuous subcutaneous insulin infusion in neonatal diabetes mellitus. Diabetologia 1999;42(suppl 1):A212.

8 Cave H, Polak M, Drunat S, Denamur E, Czernichow P: Refinement of the 6q chromosomal region implicated in transient neonatal diabetes. Diabetes 2000;49:108–113.

9 Vaxillaire M, Populaire C, Busiah K, Cave H, Gloyn AL, Hattersley AT, Czernichow P, Froguel P, Polak M: Kir6.2 mutations are a common cause of permanent neonatal diabetes in a large cohort of French patients. Diabetes 2004;53:2719–2722.

10 Babenko AP, Polak M, Cave H, Busiah K, Czernichow P, Scharfmann R, Bryan J, Aguilar-Bryan L, Vaxillaire M, Froguel P: Activating mutations in the ABCC8 gene in neonatal diabetes mellitus. N Engl J Med 2006;355:456–466.

11 Vaxillaire M, Dechaume A, Busiah K, Cave H, Pereira S, Scharfmann R, de Nanclares GP, Castano L, Froguel P, Polak M, SUR1-Neonatal Diabetes Study Group: New ABCC8 mutations in relapsing neonatal diabetes and clinical features. Diabetes 2007;56:1737–1741.

Dr. Nadia Tubiana-Rufi
Department of Endocrinology and Diabetology
Robert Debré Hospital, AP-HP, 48 bd Serurier
FR–75019 Paris (France)
Tel. +33 1 40 03 23 60, Fax +33 1 40 03 24 29, E-Mail nadia.tubiana@rdb.aphp.fr

Shield JPH, Scharfmann R (eds): Development of the Pancreas and Neonatal Diabetes.
Endocr Dev. Basel, Karger, 2007, vol 12, pp 75–85

Generating New Candidate Genes for Neonatal Diabetes: Functional and Genetic Studies of Insulin Secretion in Type 2 Diabetes

Guy A. Rutter

Department of Cell Biology, Division of Medicine, Imperial College London, London, UK

Abstract

Although the molecular lesions underlying a substantial proportion of all cases of permanent and neonatal diabetes have now been defined, in as many as 30% of cases the defect is unknown. Three complementary approaches may help to define further disease-causing changes: (1) the molecular dissection of the insulin secretory process itself using cellular, physiological and imaging techniques; (2) measurements of the level of expression of β-cell genes in islets from rodents or humans with type 2 diabetes (T2D) by oligonucleotide micro-array or proteomic analysis, and (3) population-wide whole-genome association studies of T2D. Here, I survey recent published data in this context.

Permanent and transient neonatal diabetes mellitus are rare disorders usually presenting in infants a few days after birth and frequently caused by chromosomal rearrangements or point mutations [see contributions from Shield, Temple, and Polak, this vol.], which lead to insulin secretory deficiencies. Whilst the underlying genomic changes are increasingly well defined, in a substantial number of cases the cause of the disease is still unclear. In this chapter, I present a brief survey of the present understanding of the mechanisms which regulate insulin secretion in the healthy β-cell. As a further means to identify candidates affected in forms of transient neonatal diabetes mellitus or permanent neonatal diabetes mellitus whose molecular aetiology is presently undefined, I then describe recent 'unbiased' approaches to identifying mis-expressed or mutated genes associated with type 2 diabetes (T2D).

Molecular Mechanisms of Nutrient-Stimulated Insulin Secretion from Pancreatic Islet β-Cells

In healthy individuals, the uptake of glucose or other nutrient secretagogues into β-cells stimulates the secretion of insulin chiefly by enhancing oxidative metabolism and ATP synthesis [1]. Closure of ATP-sensitive K^+ channels (K_{ATP}) on the plasma membrane then leads to cellular depolarisation, the opening of voltage-sensitive L-type Ca^{2+} channels [2] and the triggered exocytosis of insulin from large dense-core vesicles (LDCVs) [3]. Further 'K_{ATP}-independent' or 'amplifying' mechanisms of glucose action [4, 5] may also sensitise the secretory machinery to changes in cytosolic free [Ca^{2+}] ($[Ca^{2+}]_c$). The latter may then drive the recruitment of LDCVs from a reserve to a readily releasable pool [6], and contribute to a sustained or 'second phase' of insulin release [1, 7]. The mechanisms involved in this amplifying phase are still very poorly understood but possibly involve the generation of glutamate [8, 9], citrate [10], or NADPH [11, 12], as well as enhanced Ca^{2+} influx through R-type Ca^{2+} channels [13] or the inhibition of AMP-activated protein kinase (AMPK) [14–18].

Physiological potentiators of insulin secretion including acetylcholine [19], which contribute to the cephalic phase of insulin release [20], and the enteric factor glucagon-like peptide 1 (GLP-1) [21, 22], which enhances insulin secretion postabsorptively, act at least in part to mobilise intracellular [Ca^{2+}]. In the former case, this involves the activation of phospholipase C, generation of inositol 1,4,5 trisphosphate and the release of calcium from the endoplasmic reticulum (ER). The means through which GLP-1 affects intracellular [Ca^{2+}] in β-cells are more complex but appear to involve increases in the cAMP level and the engagement of the guanine nucleotide exchange factor, Epac (exchange protein activated by cAMP). Rap, a low-molecular-weight GTPase of the Ras superfamily [23], and ryanodine receptors [24] are then likely to mediate Ca^{2+} release from the ER or other stores [22, 25], potentially including LDCVs [26]. The consequent increase in $[Ca^{2+}]_c$ may, in turn, stimulate mitochondrial ATP synthesis [22] causing closure of K_{ATP} channels, and calcium influx in a feed-forward loop. Release of Ca^{2+} from intracellular stores [27] may also modulate the activation of secretion by glucose [28] both directly and through the control of plasma membrane potential [29, 30].

Evidence for the crucial role in β-cell glucose/nutrient sensing of K_{ATP} channels is overwhelming, and derives both from cellular studies [31] and from recent human data from human genetics (see also below). Notably, mutations in both *KCNJ11,* encoding Kir6.2 [32] and *ABCC8,* encoding SUR1 [33, 34], have been linked to transient and permanent neonatal diabetes and explain close to 50% of all cases of diabetes presenting at age <6 months. However, K_{ATP} channels are not the only glucose sensors; the whole metabolic configuration of the β-cell is set up to allow changes in glucose concentrations over the physiological range to enhance oxidative metabolism. In addition to the expression of the low-affinity glucose transporter Glut2 [35] and glucokinase [36] as pivotal glucose sensors, β-cells express remarkably low levels of both lactate dehydrogenase [37–39] and the plasma membrane lactate/pyruvate transporter, MCT-1, encoded by *SLC16A1* [40], and ubiquitously expressed at high levels in the majority of other tissues. Overexpression of MCT-1 reduces glucose-induced insulin secretion [41] and permits stimulation of release in response to pyruvate [42]. We have recently shown that mutations in the promoter regions of the corresponding gene, *SLC16A1,* are linked to exercise-induced hyperinsulinism [43], demonstrating the importance of low MCT-1 levels also in man in preventing the inappropriate stimulation of insulin secretion during exercise. Whether polymorphisms in the *SLC16A1* gene are also associated with the development of diabetes, due to abnormal glucose sensing, remains to be determined.

Both human genetics and approaches using rodent models have also revealed possible new genes which might be linked to neonatal diabetes. Thus, imaging of individual secretory events at the single-cell level [44, 45] has shown that individual interactions between the vesicle and plasma membrane, and the opening of a fusion pore, vary considerably in their nature and duration. Importantly, shorter fusion events, and more limited release of insulin, were observed in rat β-cells cultured for 24 h in the presence of high glucose concentrations. Examined in diabetic human β-cells [46], Zucker diabetic fatty rat β-cells [47] and INS1 cells [48, 49], high glucose (and high lipid levels; 'glucolipotoxity') is associated with decreases in the expression of genes involved in the exocytotic process, notably SNARE (soluble N-ethylmaleimide-sensitive fusion attachment receptor) proteins including SNAP25 and syntaxin, as well as Rab3, Rab27a, VAMP2, synaptotagmin V and RIM-binding protein, possibly due to an increase in cAMP levels and activation of the transcriptional repressor CREM/ICER [48]. By contrast, levels of dynamin 1, which appears to terminate each release event [50], are unchanged, possibly slowing the exoytotic process relative to vesicle recapture ('cavity recapture') [50].

Type 2 Diabetes Genes: Micro-Array and Whole-Genome Association Studies

T2D currently afflicts about 6% of the population of westernised societies and usually involves both insulin resistance and inadequate pancreatic insulin production [51]. The latter deficit appears to result from severely abnormal triggering of insulin release from the extant β-cell mass [52] confounded by defective maintenance or expansion of β-cell numbers [53].

A small proportion of T2D cases belong to a class of monogenic disorders (maturity-onset diabetes of the young) [54], and mutations in some of the genes involved (notably *IPF1, GCK* and *HNF1β;* see below) are also observed in some cases (<4%) of neonatal diabetes. There is little doubt that the more common forms of T2D also have a strong genetic component, with the risk of the disease elevated by approximately 3.5-fold between first-degree relatives, whilst concordance between monozygotic twins is about 80% [55]. Thus, an interaction between environmental factors, including an obesogenic westernised diet and sedentary lifestyle, and an at-risk genetic predisposition, probably involving many genes, seems likely to explain the majority of T2D cases.

Although the precise nature of the defects at the tissue level is disputed, both insulin resistance and β-cell failure undoubtedly play a role in T2D, with the critical contribution of the latter having only been recognised in recent years. Whether decreases in β-cell mass (as observed in type 1 diabetes) or function are the chief defect in T2D is also a matter of debate. Recent studies [53] demonstrated decreases of as much as 40% in β-cell mass after death in pancreata from T2D patients compared to age- and weight-matched controls. On the other hand, many studies down the years have shown a clear loss of β-cell responsiveness to glucose, both in terms of metabolism and secretion [52, 56, 57], thus convincingly illustrating a functional defect in the existing β-cells. Moreover, whilst decreases in pancreatic endocrine cells were seen during development of transgenic mice carrying the imprinted ZAC locus from human 6q24 and associated with transient neonatal diabetes, β-cell mass was normal or elevated at all stages after birth [58], pointing to a functional defect in this model.

Likewise, genetic studies have highlighted associations with genes likely to be involved in regulating insulin release acutely, including *GCK*, the K_{ATP} channel subunits Kir6.2 *(KCNJ11)* [32], SUR1 *(ABCC8)* [34], as well as transcription factors such as HNF4α, implicated in the maintenance of mitochondrial metabolism [59], and PPARγ [60]. Very recent whole-genome association studies [61–64] (table 1) have demonstrated the key importance of genes whose products are essential for insulin accumulation into dense-core granules *(SLC30A8; ZnT-8)* [65], and β-cell function, but also those implicated in β-cell proliferation or growth. These include, notably, *TCF7L2,* the human homologue of TCF4 in mice which was also identified in earlier association studies [66], and HHEX, both of whose products are involved in signalling downstream of *wnt* receptors (see below). Other genes include those involved in the regulation of the cell cycle such as the cyclin-dependent kinases CDKAL1 and CDK2N1 [64]. Interestingly, *TCF7L2* mRNA levels were *raised* in our micro-array analysis of islets from a rodent model of T2D, the Zucker diabetic fatty rat [47], though whether this change represents a causative event or part of a compensatory mechanism in this model remains to be clarified. This study also revealed decreases in the expression of Pdx1 and MafA, genes involved in the development and differentiated function of β-cells, which were corrected by overexpression of a dominant-negative form of the lipogenic transcription factor SREBP1c. This observation suggested that the above changes may result at least in part from 'glucolipotoxic' effects on the β-cells in this model of obesity-induced diabetes. On the other hand, SREBP1c suppression did not affect the abnormalities in the expression of other key developmental genes including Pax6, Arx, HNF1α, and HNF3β/Foxa2, inducible cyclic AMP early repressor implicating the latter as more fundamental to the secretory phenotype in this setting. Similar results were also obtained in a micro-array-based study of human

Table 1. Genome-wide scan for human T2D genes

SNP	Chromosome	Position	Gene	Stage 1	Stage 2	Combined
rs7903146	10	114748339	TCF7L2	3.94×10^{-19}	1.51×10^{-34}	9.70×10^{-52}
rs13266634	8	118253964	SLC30A8	7.18×10^{-6}	6.15×10^{-8}	2.14×10^{-11}
rs1111875	10	94452862	HHEX	2.58×10^{-6}	2.96×10^{-6}	3.74×10^{-10}
rs7923837	10	94471897		8.58×10^{-7}	7.53×10^{-6}	4.57×10^{-10}
rs2876711	13	76314505		9.34×10^{-6}	1.41×10^{-3}	1.93×10^{-6}
rs3740878	11	44214378	EXT2	7.18×10^{-6}	1.17×10^{-4}	2.42×10^{-6}
rs10823406	10	70982029		1.12×10^{-5}	2.65×10^{-3}	6.36×10^{-6}
rs6413504	19	11102915	LDLR	2.65×10^{-5}	2.78×10^{-3}	9.14×10^{-6}
rs1193179	1	7503868	CAMTA1	3.96×10^{-7}	9.06×10^{-3}	1.24×10^{-5}
rs729287	11	44236666		9.01×10^{-6}	6.71×10^{-4}	1.64×10^{-5}
rs2499953	11	4967481	MMP26	9.41×10^{-6}	7.04×10^{-3}	1.83×10^{-5}
rs1256517	14	64805437		2.51×10^{-5}	5.12×10^{-3}	2.40×10^{-5}
rs1005316	17	66501964		9.57×10^{-6}	8.31×10^{-4}	2.13×10^{-4}
rs282705	4	59343615		2.82×10^{-6}	1.46×10^{-1}	5.35×10^{-4}
rs8101509	19	57100638	FLJ12644	7.76×10^{-6}	1.00×10^{-1}	6.23×10^{-4}
rs2589001	16	53776363		2.73×10^{-6}	9.85×10^{-2}	6.51×10^{-4}
rs10483096	22	16926334	PEX26	1.40×10^{-5}	1.02×10^{-1}	7.74×10^{-4}

Note that TCF7L2 and HHEX are involved in Wnt/β-catenin signalling and are likely to contribute to β-cell development. SLC30A8 encodes an islet cell secretory vesicle-specific zinc transporter. See the text for other details. Modified from Sladek et al. [61].

islets from control versus T2D patients [67], revealing changes in the expression of signalling molecules downstream of the insulin and insulin-like growth factor receptors (IRS2, PKB/Akt2), consistent with the importance of this signalling pathway in normal β-cell development and function [68–70], as well as HNF4α and aryl hydrocarbon receptor nuclear translocator (ARNT) also called hypoxia-inducible factor 1β. Inactivation of the latter, a member of the basic helix-loop-helix Per/AhR/ARNT/Sim transcription factor family essential in embryonic development [71], in β-cells led to defective insulin secretion and abnormal glucose tolerance in knockout mice [67].

The above results point to a crucial requirement either for the establishment of adequate numbers of β-cell precursors in early development, or for the capacity for β-cell replication [72] when demanded under diabetogenic conditions, such as to supply increased insulin demand as a result of peripheral insulin resistance. Thus, in the absence of treatment, carriers of the at-risk TT allele of *TCF7L2* had an increased risk of diabetes of close to 50% 4 years after disease onset compared to controls hetero- or homozygous for the control (C) allele; smaller, but still significant differences were also observed for disease progression in patients treated with diet/exercise or metformin [73]. It is perhaps notable then that *TCF7L2* lies at the end of the *wnt*/β-catenin pathway, recently implicated in β-cell growth or development [74, 75], and which acts by up-regulating transcription factors involved in cell cycle control.

TCF7L2 is expressed ubiquitously in mammalian tissues including (in contrast to an early report [76]) pancreatic islet β-cells [77]. Mice homozygous for deletion of *TCF7L2* inactivation die just after birth and lack gut L-cell precursors [78]. This observation has implicated defective GLP-1 release in the aetiology of diabetes in affected individuals. However, at the time of writing, differences in serum GLP-1 levels between CC and TT individuals have not been reported. By contrast, this laboratory has observed that silencing of *TCF7L2* expression by RNA interference in either MIN6 or INS1 (832/13) β-cells [79] reduces both basal and glucose-stimulated insulin secretion, whilst having minimal if any effect on prepro-insulin gene expression or total insulin levels. The molecular basis of such an effect on the acute actions of glucose remains to be defined. Likewise, the mechanisms through which the disease-associated mutations affect TCF7L2 at the protein level require further study.

SLC30A8 encodes ZnT-8, a pancreatic β-cell (and possibly α-cell) restricted transporter of zinc ions into secretory vesicles. The T2D-associated non-synonymous polymorphism [61] results in the replacement of arginine at position 325 with a tryptophan. Although a high-resolution crystal structure for ZnT-8 is presently unavailable, preliminary modelling studies suggest that R325, which interestingly is not concerned in the rodent sequence, lies in a loop close to a zinc-binding domain, such that its mutation may reduce the binding effect and hence the transport kinetics for zinc uptake into the granule.

Other Candidate β-Cell Genes: The Nutrient-Regulated Protein Kinases AMP-Activated Protein Kinase and Per-Arnt-Sim Kinase

AMPK is an evolutionarily conserved fuel-sensitive protein kinase, stimulated by low levels of nutrients, and an increase in AMP/ATP concentration ratio [80, 81]. The heterotrimeric enzyme comprises a catalytic α-subunit encoded by one of two genes (α_1, α_2), a scaffold β-subunit (β_1 or β_2) and an AMP-binding regulator subunit (γ_1, γ_2, or γ_3) [80, 81]. Activation of AMPK is associated with phosphorylation of the α-subunit at Thr-172 by upstream kinases such as LKB1 [82]. Activation of AMPK in the liver in response to antihyperglycaemic agents such as metformin [83] or thiazolidinediones [84] reduces hepatic glucose production [83] by a TORC2-mediated decrease in gluconeogenic gene expression [85]. In the β-cell, by contrast, AMPK activity is 'constitutively' elevated at low (physiologically fasting) glucose concentrations [15, 16, 86] but is reduced as glucose concentrations rise, suggesting a role for the enzyme in the regulation of insulin secretion. Correspondingly, when the inhibition of AMPK is prevented by expression of a constitutively activated (T172D) form of the enzyme [87], insulin secretion is substantially blocked [16]. Whilst the molecular mechanisms through which AMPK controls secretion need to be fully defined, reduced movement of secretory granules [17] and an inhibitory phosphorylation of kinesin light chains [3] may be involved, as well as phosphorylation of acetyl-CoA carboxylase, and activation of fatty acid oxidation [16].

Further supporting a role for AMPK phosphorylation in the β-cell in vivo, expression of activated AMPK reduced the ability of transplanted islets to reverse streptozotocin-induced diabetes in mice [18]; data on transgenic mice overexpressing dominant-negative or active AMPK selectively in β-cells and further investigation of the role of other members of the stress-activated family of proteins including per-arnt-sim kinase (PASK) [88] are eagerly awaited. The role of the latter is particularly intriguing: unlike AMPK, PASK activity and expression are both increased in islets and clonal β-cells as glucose levels rise [88], and PASK silencing decreases the expression of key β-cell genes including *Pdx1* and prepro-insulin. Moreover, mice inactivated for both PASK alleles display glucose intolerance and defective insulin secretion [J. Rutter, University of Utah, unpubl. results]. PASK is an intriguing target for therapeutic intervention, since the PAS domain represents a potential drug binding site [89]. Moreover, we have recently identified mutations in the catalytic kinase domain which are associated with familial T2D [M. Vaxillaire, unpubl. obs.] suggesting that mutations in this gene may lead to defective insulin secretion and might contribute to other forms of the disease, including neonatal diabetes.

Concluding Remarks

A battery of classical cell biological approaches has been combined in recent years with 'high density', unbiased screening approaches for changes in the expression of genes, as well as for disease-associated polymorphisms, which may enhance the risk of T2D. An intriguing, if unexpected observation has been that the genes identified through population-based screens are, almost without exception, associated with the secretion rather than the action of insulin. Whilst still being far from providing confident disease prediction [90], the identified genes have generated a wealth of new targets for therapeutic intervention in T2D and, given their likely role in regulating β-cell function, several are possible candidates as neonatal diabetes genes. Future studies with affected patients should allow some of the best candidates to be tested.

Acknowledgements

This study was supported by Wellcome Trust Programme Grants (067081/Z/02/Z, 081958/Z/07/Z), and grants from the NIH (RO1 DK071962-01), MRC (G0401641), Diabetes UK (RD04/0002895) and European Union FP6 ('Save beta').

References

1 Rutter GA: Visualising insulin secretion. The Minkowski Lecture 2004. Diabetologia 2004;47: 1861–1872.

2 Safayhi H, Haase H, Kramer U, Bihlmayer A, Roenfeldt M, Ammon HPT, Froschmayr M, Cassidy TN, Morano I, et al: L-Type calcium channels in insulin-secreting cells: biochemical characterization and phosphorylation in RINm5F cells. Mol Endocrinol 1997;11:619–629.

3 Rutter GA, Hill EV: Insulin vesicle release: walk, kiss, pause ... then run. Physiology (Bethesda) 2006; 21:189–196.

4 Henquin JC: Triggering and amplifying pathways of regulation of insulin secretion by glucose. Diabetes 2000;49:1751–1760.

5 Komatsu M, Schermerhorn T, Noda M, Straub SG, Aizawa T, Sharp GG: Augmentation of insulin release by glucose in the absence of extracellular Ca^{2+}: new insights into stimulus-secretion coupling. Diabetes 1997;46:1928–1938.

6 Varadi A, Ainscow EK, Allan VJ, Rutter GA: Involvement of conventional kinesin in glucose-stimulated secretory granule movements and exocytosis in clonal pancreatic β-cells. J Cell Sci 2002;115: 4177–4189.

7 Rorsman P, Renstrom E: Insulin granule dynamics in pancreatic beta cells. Diabetologia 2003;46: 1029–1045.

8 Maechler P, Wollheim CB: Mitochondrial glutamate acts as a messenger in glucose-induced insulin exocytosis. Nature 1999;402:685–689.

9 Eto K, Yamashita T, Hirose K, Tsubamoto Y, Ainscow EK, Rutter GA, Kimura S, Noda M, Iino M, et al: Glucose metabolism and glutamate analog acutely alkalinize pH of insulin secretory vesicles of pancreatic beta-cells. Am J Physiol Endocrinol Metab 2003;285:E262–E271.

10 Farfari S, Schulz V, Corkey B, Prentki M: Glucose-regulated anaplerosis and cataplerosis in pancreatic beta-cells: possible implication of a pyruvate/citrate shuttle in insulin secretion. Diabetes 2000;49:718–726.

11 Ronnebaum SM, Ilkayeva O, Burgess SC, Joseph JW, Lu D, Stevens RD, Becker TC, Sherry AD, Newgard CB, et al: A pyruvate cycling pathway involving cytosolic NADP-dependent isocitrate dehydrogenase regulates glucose-stimulated insulin secretion. J Biol Chem 2006;281:30593–30602.

12 Ivarsson R, Quintens R, Dejonghe S, Tsukamoto K, in 't Veld P, Renstrom E, Schuit FC: Redox control of exocytosis: regulatory role of NADPH, thioredoxin, and glutaredoxin. Diabetes 2005;54:2132–2142.

13 Schulla V, Renstrom E, Feil R, Feil S, Franklin I, Gjinovci A, Jing XJ, Laux D, Lundquist I, et al: Impaired insulin secretion and glucose tolerance in beta cell-selective Ca(v)1.2 Ca^{2+} channel null mice. EMBO J 2003;22:3844–3854.

14 Salt I, Celler JW, Hawley SA, Prescott A, Woods A, Carling D, Hardie DG: AMP-activated protein kinase: greater AMP dependence, and preferential nuclear localization, of complexes containing the alpha2 isoform. Biochem J 1998;334:177–187.

15 Da Silva Xavier G, Leclerc I, Salt IP, Doiron B, Hardie DG, Kahn A, Rutter GA: Role of AMP-activated protein kinase in the regulation by glucose of islet beta-cell gene expression. Proc Natl Acad Sci USA 2000;97:4023–4028.

16 Da Silva Xavier G, Leclerc I, Varadi A, Tsuboi T, Moule SK, Rutter GA: Role for AMP-activated protein kinase in glucose-stimulated insulin secretion and preproinsulin gene expression. Biochem J 2003; 371:761–774.

17 Tsuboi T, da Silva Xavier G, Leclerc I, Rutter GA: 5′-AMP-activated protein kinase controls insulin-containing secretory vesicle dynamics. J Biol Chem 2003;278:52042–52051.

18 Richards SK, Parton LE, Leclerc I, Rutter GA, Smith RM: Overexpression of AMP-activated protein kinase impairs pancreatic beta-cell function in vivo. J Endocrinol 2005;187:225–235.

19 Wollheim CB, Biden TJ: Signal transduction in insulin secretion: comparison between fuel stimuli and receptor agonists. Ann NY Acad Sci 1986;488: 317–333.

20 Ahren B, Holst JJ: The cephalic insulin response to meal ingestion in humans is dependent on both cholinergic and noncholinergic mechanisms and is important for postprandial glycemia. Diabetes 2001;50:1030–1038.

21 Nauck MA, Holst JJ, Willms B, Schmiegel W: Glucagon-like peptide 1 (GLP-1) as a new therapeutic approach for type 2-diabetes. Exp Clin Endocrinol Diabetes 1997;105:187–195.

22 Tsuboi T, da Silva Xavier G, Holz GG, Jouaville LS, Thomas AP, Rutter GA: Glucagon-like peptide-1 mobilizes intracellular Ca^{2+} and stimulates mitochondrial ATP synthesis in pancreatic MIN6 beta-cells. Biochem J 2003;369:287–299.

23 Reuther GW, Der CJ: The Ras branch of small GTPases: Ras family members don't fall far from the tree. Curr Opin Cell Biol 2000;12:157–165.

24 Islam MS: The ryanodine receptor calcium channel of beta-cells: molecular regulation and physiological significance. Diabetes 2002;51:1299–1309.

25 Holz GG: Epac: A new cAMP-binding protein in support of glucagon-like peptide-1 receptor-mediated signal transduction in the pancreatic beta-cell. Diabetes 2004;53:5–13.
26 Mitchell KJ, Lai FA, Rutter GA: Ryanodine receptor type I and nicotinic acid adenine dinucleotide phosphate (NAADP) receptors mediate Ca^{2+} release from insulin-containing vesicles in living pancreatic beta-cells (MIN6). J Biol Chem 2003; 278:11057–11064.
27 Rutter GA, Tsuboi T: Kiss and run exocytosis of dense core secretory vesicles. Neuroreport 2004;15: 79–81.
28 Rutter GA, Tsuboi T, Ravier MA: Ca^{2+} microdomains and the control of insulin secretion. Cell Calcium 2006;40:539–551.
29 Gilon P, Arredouani A, Gailly P, Gromada J, Henquin JC: Uptake and release of Ca^{2+} by the endoplasmic reticulum contribute to the oscillations of the cytosolic Ca^{2+} concentration triggered by Ca^{2+} influx in the electrically excitable pancreatic β-cell. J Biol Chem 1999;274:20197–20205.
30 Mitchell KJ, Tsuboi T, Rutter GA: Role for plasma membrane-related Ca^{2+}-ATPase-1 (PMR1/ATP2C1) in pancreatic β-cell Ca^{2+} homeostasis revealed by RNA silencing. Diabetes 2004;53:393–400.
31 Ashcroft F, Rorsman P: Type 2 diabetes mellitus: not quite exciting enough? Hum Mol Genet 2004; 13:R21–R31.
32 Gloyn AL, Pearson ER, Antcliff JF, Proks P, Bruining GJ, Slingerland AS, Howard N, Srinivasan S, Silva JM, et al: Activating mutations in the gene encoding the ATP-sensitive potassium-channel subunit Kir6.2 and permanent neonatal diabetes. N Engl J Med 2004;350:1838–1849.
33 Proks P, Arnold AL, Bruining J, Girard C, Flanagan SE, Larkin B, Colclough K, Hattersley AT, Ashcroft FM, et al: A heterozygous activating mutation in the sulphonylurea receptor SUR1 (ABCC8) causes neonatal diabetes. Hum Mol Genet 2006;15:1793–1800.
34 Babenko AP, Polak M, Cave H, Busiah K, Czernichow P, Scharfmann R, Bryan J, Guilar-Bryan L, Vaxillaire M, et al: Activating mutations in the ABCC8 gene in neonatal diabetes mellitus. N Engl J Med 2006;355:456–466.
35 Thorens B, Sarkar HK, Kaback HR, Lodish HF: Cloning and functional expression in bacteria of a novel glucose transporter present in liver intestine kidney and β-pancreatic islet cells. Cell 1988;55: 281–290.
36 Iynedjian PB: Mammalian glucokinase and its gene. Biochem J 1993;293:1–13.
37 Sekine N, Cirulli V, Regazzi R, Brown LJ, Gine E, Tamarit-Rodriguez J, Girotti M, Marie S, MacDonald MJ, et al: Low lactate dehydrogenase and high mitochondrial glycerol phosphate dehydrogenase in pancreatic β-cell. Potential role in nutrient sensing. J Biol Chem 1994;269:4895–4902.
38 Liang Y, Bai G, Doliba N, Buettger C, Wang L, Berner DK, Matschinsky FM: Glucose metabolism and insulin release in mouse beta HC9 cells, as model for wild-type pancreatic beta-cells. Am J Physiol 1996;270:E846–E857.
39 Schuit F, DeVos A, Farfari S, Moens K, Pipeleers D, Brun T, Prentki M: Metabolic fate of glucose in purified islet cells – Glucose-regulated anaplerosis in beta cells. J Biol Chem 1997;272:18572–18579.
40 Zhao C, Wilson CM, Schuit F, Halestrap AP, Rutter GA: Expression and distribution of lactate/monocarboxylate transporter (MCT) isoforms in pancreatic islets and the exocrine pancreas. Diabetes 2001; 50:361–366.
41 Zhao C, Rutter GA: Overexpression of lactate dehydrogenase A attenuates glucose-induced insulin secretion in stable MIN-6 beta-cell lines. FEBS Lett 1998;430:213–216.
42 Ishihara H, Wang H, Drewes LR, Wollheim CB: Overexpression of monocarboxylate transporter and lactate dehydrogenase alters insulin secretory responses to pyruvate and lactate in beta cells. J Clin Invest 1999;104:1621–1629.
43 Otonkoski T, et al: Physical exercise-induced hyperinsulinemic hypoglycemia caused by failure of monocarboxylate transporter 1 silencing in pancreatic beta cells. Am J Hum Genet, in press.
44 Tsuboi T, Rutter GA: Multiple forms of 'kiss-and-run' exocytosis revealed by evanescent wave microscopy. Curr Biol 2003;13:563–567.
45 Tsuboi T, Ravier MA, Parton LE, Rutter GA: Sustained exposure to elevated glucose concentrations modifies glucose signalling and the mechanics of secretory vesicle fusion in primary rat pancreatic β-cells. Diabetes 2006;55:1057–1065.
46 Ostenson CG, Gaisano H, Sheu L, Tibell A, Bartfai T: Impaired gene and protein expression of exocytotic soluble N-ethylmaleimide attachment protein receptor complex proteins in pancreatic islets of type 2 diabetic patients. Diabetes 2006;55:435–440.
47 Parton LE, McMillen PJ, Shen Y, Docherty E, Sharpe E, Diraison F, Briscoe CP, Rutter GA: Limited role for SREBP-1c in defective glucose-induced insulin secretion from Zucker diabetic fatty rat islets: a functional and gene profiling analysis. Am J Physiol Endocrinol Metab 2006;291:E982–E994.
48 Abderrahmani A, Cheviet S, Ferdaoussi M, Coppola T, Waeber G, Regazzi R: ICER induced by hyperglycemia represses the expression of genes essential for insulin exocytosis. EMBO J 2006;25: 977–986.

49 Dubois M, Vacher P, Roger B, Huyghe D, Vandewalle B, Kerr-Conte J, Pattou F, Moustaid-Moussa N, Lang J: Glucotoxicity inhibits late steps of insulin exocytosis. Endocrinology 2007;148:1605–1614.
50 Tsuboi T, McMahon HT, Rutter GA: Mechanisms of dense core vesicle recapture following 'kiss and run' ('cavicapture') exocytosis in insulin-secreting cells. J Biol Chem 2004;279:47115–47124.
51 Zimmet P, Alberti KG, Shaw J: Global and societal implications of the diabetes epidemic. Nature 2001; 414:782–787.
52 Del Guerra S, Lupi R, Marselli L, Masini M, Bugliani M, Sbrana S, Torri S, Pollera M, Boggi U, et al: Functional and molecular defects of pancreatic islets in human type 2 diabetes. Diabetes 2005;54: 727–735.
53 Butler AE, Janson J, Bonner-Weir S, Ritzel R, Rizza RA, Butler PC: Beta-cell deficit and increased beta-cell apoptosis in humans with type 2 diabetes. Diabetes 2003;52:102–110.
54 Hattersley AT: Maturity-onset diabetes of the young: clinical heterogeneity explained by genetic heterogeneity. Diabet Med 1998;15:15–24.
55 Barnett AH, Spiliopoulos AJ, Pyke DA, Stubbs WA, Burrin J, Alberti KG: Metabolic studies in unaffected co-twins of non-insulin-dependent diabetics. Br Med J (Clin Res Ed) 1981;282:1656–1658.
56 Fernandez-Alvarez J, Conget I, Rasschaert J, Sener A, Gomis R, Malaisse WJ: Enzymatic, metabolic and secretory patterns in human islets of type 2 (non-insulin-dependent) diabetic patients. Diabetologia 1994;37:177–181.
57 Anello M, Lupi R, Spampinato D, Piro S, Masini M, Boggi U, Del Prato S, Rabuazzo AM, Purrello F, et al: Functional and morphological alterations of mitochondria in pancreatic beta cells from type 2 diabetic patients. Diabetologia 2005;48:282–289.
58 Ma D, Shield JP, Dean W, Leclerc I, Knauf C, Burcelin RR, Rutter GA, Kelsey G: Altered glucose homeostasis in transgenic mice expressing the human transient neonatal diabetes mellitus locus (TNDM). J Clin Invest 2004;114:339–348.
59 Gauthier BR, Brun T, Sarret EJ, Ishihara H, Schaad O, Descombes P, Wollheim CB: Oligonucleotide microarray analysis reveals PDX1 as an essential regulator of mitochondrial metabolism in rat islets. J Biol Chem 2004;279:31121–31130.
60 Hegele RA, Cao H, Harris SB, Zinman B, Hanley AJ, Anderson CM: Peroxisome proliferator-activated receptor-gamma2 P12A and type 2 diabetes in Canadian Oji-Cree. J Clin Endocrinol Metab 2000; 85:2014–2019.
61 Sladek R, Rocheleau G, Rung J, Dina C, Shen L, Serre D, Boutin P, Vincent D, Delisle A, et al: A genome-wide association study identifies novel risk loci for type 2 diabetes. Nature 2007;445:881–885.
62 Saxena R, Voight BF, Lyssenko V, Burtt NP, de Bakker PI, Chen H, Roix JJ, Kathiresan S, Hirschhorn JN, et al: Genome-wide association analysis identifies loci for type 2 diabetes and triglyceride levels. Science 2007;316:1331–1336.
63 Scott LJ, Mohlke KL, Bonnycastle LL, Willer CJ, Li Y, Duren WL, Erdos MR, Stringham HM, Chines PS, et al: A genome-wide association study of type 2 diabetes in Finns detects multiple susceptibility variants. Science 2007;316:1341–1345.
64 Zeggini E, Weedon MN, Lindgren CM, Frayling TM, Elliott KS, Lango H, Timpson NJ, Perry JR, Rayner NW, et al: Replication of genome-wide association signals in UK samples reveals risk loci for type 2 diabetes. Science 2007;316:1336–1341.
65 Chimienti F, Devergnas S, Pattou F, Schuit F, Garcia-Cuenca R, Vandewalle B, Kerr-Conte J, Van LL, Grunwald D, et al: In vivo expression and functional characterization of the zinc transporter ZnT8 in glucose-induced insulin secretion. J Cell Sci 2006; 119:4199–4206.
66 Grant SF, Thorleifsson G, Reynisdottir I, Benediktsson R, Manolescu A, Sainz J, Helgason A, Stefansson H, Emilsson V, et al: Variant of transcription factor 7-like 2 (TCF7L2) gene confers risk of type 2 diabetes. Nat Genet 2006;38:320–323.
67 Gunton JE, Kulkarni RN, Yim S, Okada T, Hawthorne WJ, Tseng YH, Roberson RS, Ricordi C, O'Connell PJ, et al: Loss of ARNT/HIF1beta mediates altered gene expression and pancreatic-islet dysfunction in human type 2 diabetes. Cell 2005; 122:337–349.
68 Kulkarni RN, Bruning JC, Winnay JN, Postic C, Magnuson MA, Kahn CR: Tissue-specific knockout of the insulin receptor in pancreatic beta cells creates an insulin secretory defect similar to that in type 2 diabetes. Cell 1999;96:329–339.
69 Leibiger IB, Leibiger B, Moede T, Berggren PO: Exocytosis of insulin promotes insulin gene transcription via the insulin receptor/PI-3 kinase/p70 s6 kinase and CaM kinase pathways. Mol Cell 1998; 1:933–938.
70 Da Silva Xavier G, Qian Q, Cullen PJ, Rutter GA: Distinct roles for insulin and insulin-like growth factor-1 receptors in pancreatic beta-cell glucose sensing revealed by RNA silencing. Biochem J 2004; 377:149–158.
71 Abbott BD, Buckalew AR: Placental defects in ARNT-knockout conceptus correlate with localized decreases in VEGF-R2, Ang-1, and Tie-2. Dev Dyn 2000;219:526–538.
72 Dor Y, Brown J, Martinez OI, Melton DA: Adult pancreatic beta-cells are formed by self-duplication rather than stem-cell differentiation. Nature 2004; 429:41–46.

73 Florez JC, Jablonski KA, Bayley N, Pollin TI, de Bakker PI, Shuldiner AR, Knowler WC, Nathan DM, Altshuler D: TCF7L2 polymorphisms and progression to diabetes in the Diabetes Prevention Program. N Engl J Med 2006;355:241–250.
74 Rulifson IC, Karnik SK, Heiser PW, ten BD, Chen H, Gu X, Taketo MM, Nusse R, Hebrok M, et al: Wnt signaling regulates pancreatic beta cell proliferation. Proc Natl Acad Sci USA 2007;104:6247–6252.
75 Dessimoz J, Bonnard C, Huelsken J, Grapin-Botton A: Pancreas-specific deletion of beta-catenin reveals Wnt-dependent and Wnt-independent functions during development. Curr Biol 2005;15:1677–1683.
76 Yi F, Brubaker PL, Jin T: TCF-4 mediates cell type-specific regulation of proglucagon gene expression by beta-catenin and glycogen synthase kinase-3beta. J Biol Chem 2005;280:1457–1464.
77 Cauchi S, Meyre D, Dina C, Choquet H, Samson C, Gallina S, Balkau B, Charpentier G, Pattou F, et al: Transcription factor TCF7L2 genetic study in the French population: expression in human beta-cells and adipose tissue and strong association with type 2 diabetes. Diabetes 2006;55:2903–2908.
78 Korinek V, Barker N, Moerer P, van Donselaar E, Huls G, Peters PJ, Clevers H: Depletion of epithelial stem-cell compartments in the small intestine of mice lacking Tcf-4. Nat Genet 1998;19:379–383.
79 Da Silva Xavier G, Rutter GA: TCF7L2 regulates glucose-stimulated insulin secretion and insulin gene expression in MIN6 β-cells. Diabetes (abstract), in press.
80 Hardie DG, Carling D, Carlson M: The AMP-activated/SNF1 protein kinase subfamily: metabolic sensors of the eukaryotic cell? Annu Rev Biochem 1998;67:821–855.
81 Rutter GA, da Silva Xavier G, Leclerc I: Roles of 5′-AMP-activated protein kinase (AMPK) in mammalian glucose homoeostasis. Biochem J 2003;375: 1–16.
82 Shaw RJ, Kosmatka M, Bardeesy N, Hurley RL, Witters LA, De Pinho RA, Cantley LC: The tumor suppressor LKB1 kinase directly activates AMP-activated kinase and regulates apoptosis in response to energy stress. Proc Natl Acad Sci USA 2004;101: 3329–3335.
83 Zhou G, Myers R, Li Y, Chen Y, Shen X, Fenyk-Melody J, Wu M, Ventre J, Doebber T, et al: Role of AMP-activated protein kinase in mechanism of metformin action. J Clin Invest 2001;108:1167–1174.
84 Fryer LG, Parbu-Patel A, Carling D: The anti-diabetic drugs rosiglitazone and metformin stimulate AMP-activated protein kinase through distinct signaling pathways. J Biol Chem 2002;277:25226–25232.
85 Koo SH, Flechner L, Qi L, Zhang X, Screaton RA, Jeffries S, Hedrick S, Xu W, Boussouar F, et al: The CREB coactivator TORC2 is a key regulator of fasting glucose metabolism. Nature 2005;437:1109–1111.
86 Salt IP, Johnson G, Ashcroft SJ, Hardie DG: AMP-activated protein kinase is activated by low glucose in cell lines derived from pancreatic beta cells, and may regulate insulin release. Biochem J 1998;335: 533–539.
87 Woods A, Azzout-Marniche D, Foretz M, Stein SC, Lemarchand P, Ferre P, Foufelle F, Carling D: Characterization of the role of AMP-activated protein kinase in the regulation of glucose-activated gene expression using constitutively active and dominant negative forms of the kinase. Mol Cell Biol 2000;20:6704–6711.
88 Da Silva Xavier G, Rutter J, Rutter GA: Involvement of Per-Arnt-Sim (PAS) kinase in the stimulation of preproinsulin and pancreatic duodenum homeobox 1 gene expression by glucose. Proc Natl Acad Sci USA 2004;101:8319–8324.
89 Rutter J, Michnoff CH, Harper SM, Gardner KH, McKnight SL: PAS kinase: an evolutionarily conserved PAS domain-regulated serine/threonine kinase. Proc Natl Acad Sci USA 2001;98:8991–8996.
90 Zeggini E, McCarthy MI: TCF7L2: the biggest story in diabetes genetics since HLA? Diabetologia 2007; 50:1–4.

Dr. Guy A. Rutter
Department of Cell Biology, Division of Medicine
Imperial College London, Sir Alexander Fleming Building
Exhibition Rd, London SW7 2AZ (UK)
Tel. +44 20 759 43340, Fax +44 20 759 43351, E-Mail g.rutter@imperial.ac.uk

Shield JPH, Scharfmann R (eds): Development of the Pancreas and Neonatal Diabetes.
Endocr Dev. Basel, Karger, 2007, vol 12, pp 86–98

Diabetes in Very Young Children and Mutations in the Insulin-Secreting Cell Potassium Channel Genes: Therapeutic Consequences

Isabelle Flechtner[a] • Martine Vaxillaire[d] • Hélène Cavé[b] • Raphael Scharfmann[c] • Philippe Froguel[d, e] • Michel Polak[a, c]

[a]Clinique des Maladies du Développement, Unité d'Endocrinologie, Diabétologie et Gynécologie Pédiatrique, Hôpital Necker-Enfants Malades, [b]Genetic biochemistry, Hôpital Robert-Debré, and [c]Unité INSERM U845, Université Paris-V, Paris, and [d]Centre National de la Recherche Scientifique UMR 8090, Institute of Biology, Pasteur Institute, Lille, France; [e]Imperial College, Hammersmith Hospital (PF), London, UK

Abstract

ATP-sensitive potassium (K_{ATP}) channels regulate the flux of K^+ ions across the cell membranes and couple cell metabolism to electrical activity. These channels are octameric complexes of 4 pore-forming Kir and 4 regulatory sulphonylurea receptor (SUR) subunits. The K_{ATP} channels play multiple physiological roles in the glucose metabolism regulation, especially in the pancreatic β-cells where they regulate insulin secretion, in response to increases in ATP concentration. Several studies have reported activating mutations in the *KCNJ11* gene, encoding the Kir6.2 subunit of the pancreatic K_{ATP} channel, in patients with permanent neonatal diabetes mellitus for 30–50% of the cases. These mutations result in reduced ATP sensitivity of the K_{ATP} channels compared with the wild types. The level of channel activity defect is responsible for different clinical features: the 'mild' form confers isolated permanent neonatal diabetes whereas the severe form combines diabetes and neurological symptoms such as epilepsy, developmental delay, muscle weakness and mild dysmorphic features. The very recently elucidated mutations in the *ABCC8* gene, encoding the second K_{ATP} channel subunit, SUR1, account for transient neonatal diabetes mellitus as well as permanent neonatal diabetes mellitus cases. In vitro studies showed no attenuation of ATP sensitivity but an increase in the opening probability of the channel through interaction of the mutated SUR1 subunit on Kir6.2. Sulphonylureas close K_{ATP} channels by binding with high affinity to SUR suggesting they could replace insulin in these patients. Subsequently, more than 60 patients have been reported as successfully switched from insulin subcutaneous injections to oral sulphonylurea therapy, with an improvement in their glycated hemoglobin. The transfer from insulin injections to oral glibenclamide therapy seems highly effective and safe for most patients, and should be performed in accordance with the legal rules for the use of such a drug, specially in children, in each country.

ATP-sensitive potassium (K_{ATP}) channels are ubiquitous channels coupling cell metabolism to electrical activity by regulating potassium movements across the cell membrane. Numerous physiological studies of these channels demonstrated their essential role in many organs, and especially in the glucose metabolism. These channels are composed of 2 types of subunits: the pore-forming Kir embraced by the regulatory sulphonylurea receptor (SUR) subunits. Several isoforms of these channels exist in different cellular types. The understanding of their role in the insulin secretion by the pancreatic β-cells and the recent identification of mutations in both subunits responsible for neonatal diabetes mellitus have opened up new therapeutic options for the patients. This review demonstrates how such advances provide an excellent example of a pharmacogenetics approach with individualization of treatment for a specific disorder.

Physiology of the ATP-Sensitive Potassium Channels

K_{ATP} channels couple cell metabolism to electrical activity by regulating potassium movement across the membrane. These channels are octameric complexes with 2 kinds of subunits: 4 regulatory SUR subunits embracing 4 pore-forming inwardly rectifying potassium channel (Kir) subunits [1, 2]. A 1:1 SUR1:KIR6.2 stoichiometry is both necessary and sufficient for assembly of active K_{ATP} channels [3, 4]. SUR, a member of the ABC transporter family, originates from 2 separate genes and therefore occurs in several spliced isoforms. SUR1 is found in the pancreatic β-cells and neurons [5], whereas SUR2A is found in heart cells and SUR2B in smooth muscle [6]. Kir6.2 subunit forms the channel pore in the majority of tissues such as pancreatic β-cell, brain, heart and skeletal muscle [3], while Kir6.1 can be found in smooth vascular muscle and astrocytes. These different channel forms have different pore properties and adenine nucleotide sensitivity [3] (fig. 1). The *KCNJ11* and *ABCC8* genes, encoding Kir6.2 and SUR1, are located at 11p15 [7], close to the large IDDM2 linkage peak.

The K_{ATP} channels play multiple physiological roles in the regulation of glucose metabolism: insulin secretion by the pancreatic β-cells, glucagon release by the pancreatic α-cells [8], somatostatin secretion from D cells [9], and GLP1 secretion from L cells [10]. When closed, the K_{ATP} channel is said to be inactivated as potassium efflux is blocked (but paradoxically this closure permits membrane depolarization and therefore the metabolic effect). Conversely, when opened, the channel is activated as potassium efflux is effective. The sulphonylurea subunits sense changes in ATP and ADP concentration and thereby affect K_{ATP} channel activity [11–13]. These nucleotides have opposite effects on the channel activity: ATP acts as a channel blocker and MgADP as a channel opener. In the pancreatic β-cells, at low glucose concentration, the potassium efflux through the opened K_{ATP} channels ('activated') sets up a membrane hyperpolarization (with a potential of about –70 mV). Increases in ATP con-

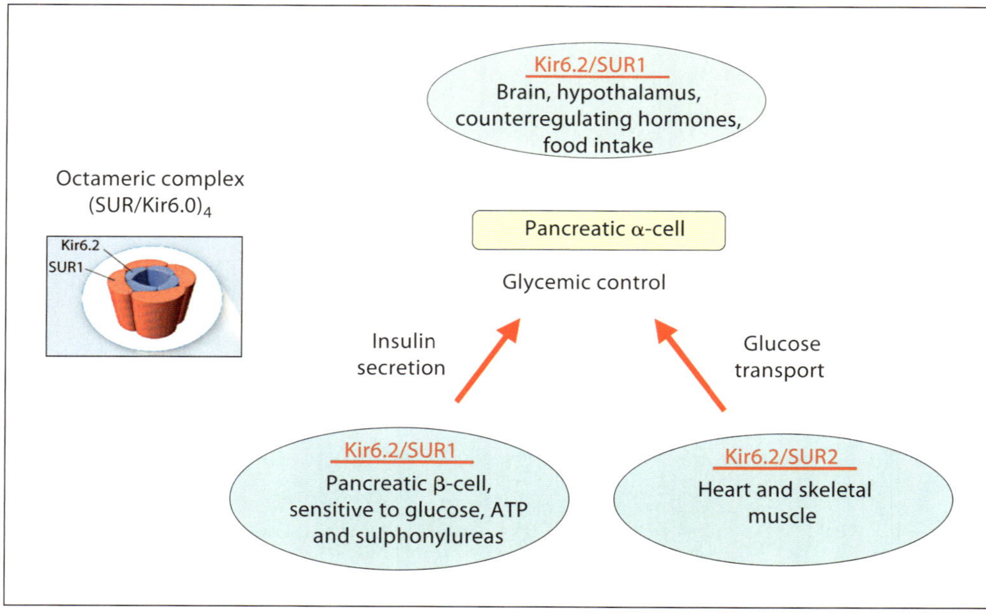

Fig. 1. Different K_{ATP} channel forms and metabolic regulation. Several isoforms of either Kir and SUR subunits are found in the different organs and confer to the channels their specificity but all interfere with the glucose metabolism. The Kir6.2/SUR1 channels are found in neurons and the pancreas, whereas the Kir6.2/SUR2 channels are found in heart and skeletal muscle.

centration (and the concomitant decrease in MgADP) in response to the glucose metabolism closes the K_{ATP} channels and is responsible for a membrane depolarization. This depolarization causes the opening of the voltage-gated Ca^{2+} channels, allowing Ca^{2+} entry triggering the exocytosis of insulin-containing granules [14] (fig. 2). Furthermore, the K_{ATP} channels are important for pancreatic insulin cell survival and regulate the differentiation of islet cells in the mice knockout for Kir6.2 [15, 16].

In cardiac, smooth and skeletal muscle and brain neuronal tissues, the K_{ATP} channels are normally closed and open in response to metabolic stress which thereby leads to inhibition of electrical activity [17]. Furthermore, studies in Kir6.1- or Kir6.2-null mice show that K_{ATP} channels are critical metabolic sensors protecting against metabolic stress such as hyper- or hypoglycemia, ischemia or hypoxia [18]. Cells expressing Kir6.2 mRNA are widely distributed throughout the brain [19] but the highest expression of K_{ATP} channels is in the substantia nigra pars reticulata which plays a pivotal role in suppressing the propagation of generalized seizures [20, 21]. The opening of K_{ATP} channels exerts a strong suppressive effect on neuronal activity during hypoxia by shifting membrane potentials in the hyperpolarized direction [22]. Mice lacking Kir6.2 are extremely susceptible to generalized seizure after brief hypoxia and K_{ATP} channels might therefore participate in a preconditioning-induced neuronal

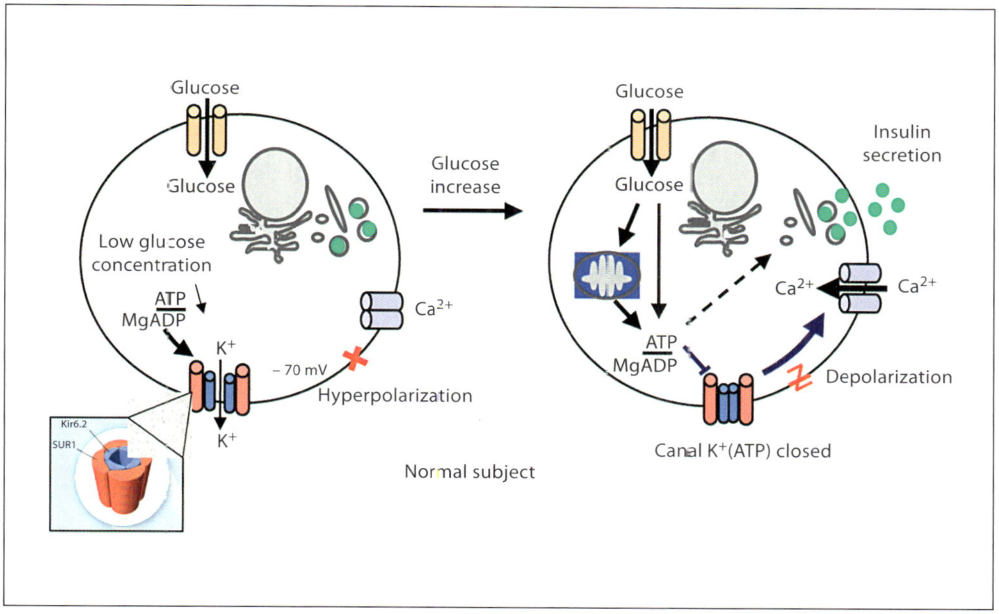

Fig. 2. K_{ATP} channels coupling cell metabolism to electrical activity in pancreatic β-cells. In the presence of low glucose and low ATP/ADP ratio, the K_{ATP} channels are opened and the cell membrane hyperpolarized. When glucose concentration and therefore ATP/ADP ratio increase, the K_{ATP} channels close, provoking membrane depolarization, opening of the voltage-gated Ca^{2+} channels and insulin exocytosis.

protection mechanism [20, 21]. Neuroglycopenia stimulates the secretion of counter-regulatory hormones, such as glucagon secretion by the pancreatic α-cells through activation of autonomic neurons. The K_{ATP} channels play a major role for glucose sensing in the ventromedial hypothalamus neurons and are impaired in the Kir6.2-null mice leading to a markedly reduced glucagon secretion [23]. Besides, in behavioral tests, the Kir6.2 knockout mice are less active, with impaired coordination and different emotional reactivity compared to the wild type, especially in novel situations [24].

In cardiac and skeletal muscle, the SUR2A isoform coexpressed with Kir6.2 is less sensitive to ATP [5]. The K_{ATP} channels link energy status of muscle fibers to the electrical activity of the cell membrane: they prevent the development of resting tension during fatigue and improve force recovery after fatigue [25]. Expressed in high density in the cardiac sarcolemma [5], K_{ATP} channels are probably associated, as in the brain, with the cardioprotective mechanism of ischemia-related preconditioning [26–29]. Under catecholamine surge, proper K_{ATP} channel activity is required for normal membrane-dependent cellular functions, such as cellular loss of potassium and adequate calcium handling [26, 27, 29, 30]. A deficit in K_{ATP} channel function in Kir6.2-null mice is recognized as a risk factor for arrhythmia under sympathetic stimulation

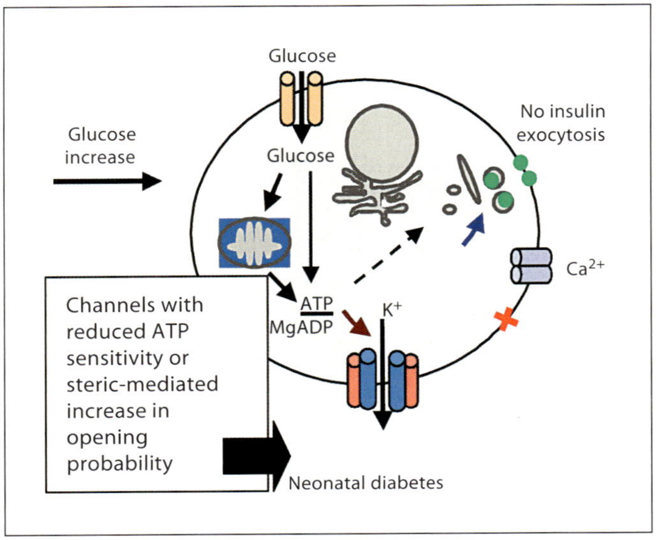

Fig. 3. Abnormal insulin secretion by *KCNJ11* or *ABCC8* activating mutations. An activating mutation is responsible for an increase in the opening probability of the channel, which inhibits the release of insulin when glucose increases.

[26, 31] and for greater susceptibility to ischemia under basal conditions [32]. However, the rapid heart rate of the mouse may magnify the relative importance of the K_{ATP} channels compared to human. Nevertheless, mutations in the cardiac SUR have been identified in patients with cardiomyopathy and ventricular arrhythmia [33]. In smooth vascular muscle, K_{ATP} channels are involved in the vessel tone [34, 35]. Two kinds of mutations have been described in Kir6.2 or SUR1 subunits. First, inactivating mutations (as in hyperinsulinism) are responsible for permanent closure of the K_{ATP} channels and therefore uncontrolled insulin exocytosis. Conversely, activating mutations (as in neonatal diabetes mellitus) provoke permanent opening of the channels and therefore membrane hyperpolarization and no insulin exocytosis.

Neonatal Diabetes due to ATP-Sensitive Potassium Channel Mutations

Large population-based cohort studies of diabetic infants suggest that early-onset permanent diabetes developing before 6 months of age differs from later-onset cases by frequent 'protective' HLA genotype for type 1 diabetes, less frequent autoimmunity and small-for-date birth weight [36]. Knowing the fundamental role of the K_{ATP} channels in the insulin secretion and the Kir6.2 mutations implied in the hyperinsulinism of infancy, mutations in Kir6.2 encoded by *KCNJ11* were searched for in type 1 and type 2 diabetes, assuming that K_{ATP} channel overactivity could cause diabetes by inhibiting insulin secretion [37] (fig. 3). Indeed, the common E23K polymorphism in Kir6.2 was found to be strongly associated with type 2 diabetes [38, 39], with decreased insulin secretion in glucose tolerance tests [40] and diminished suppression of glucagon secretion in response to hyperglycemia [41].

Thus, several studies reported sequencing of *KCNJ11,* coding for Kir6.2, in patients with permanent neonatal diabetes mellitus without known etiology (mutations in glucokinase, insulin promoter factor 1, PTF1a, FOXP3 and EIF2AK3 [42–46]) and found different mutations for 30–50% of the cases [14, 47, 48]. In our study of patients from the French Network for the Study of Neonatal Diabetes, we screened the *KCNJ11* gene in 17 term babies with a median age at diagnosis of diabetes of 64 days (range 1–260). We identified 7 heterozygous mutations in 9 patients: 3 already described (V59M, R201H, R201C) and 4 novel mutations (F35L, G53N, E322K, Y330C). Most patients had a small birth weight, probably due to in utero insulin secretory insufficiency [47]. Mutations in *KCNJ11* were also identified but with less frequency in transient neonatal diabetes cases [49]. Most of the mutations described (approximately 80% [14]) are de novo but one case has been reported with a demonstrated germ line mosaicism suggesting that this possibility should be considered when counseling recurrence risk [50]. These mutations result in reduced ATP sensitivity of the K_{ATP} channels compared with the wild types and the level of channel block is responsible for different clinical features: the 'mild' form confers isolated permanent neonatal diabetes whereas the severe form combines diabetes and neurological symptoms such as epilepsy, developmental delay, muscle weakness and mild dysmorphic features [14, 47, 48, 51]. The most frequent mutations are located in the R201 (on the C terminus) due to the presence of a CpG dinucleotide which is a hot spot mutation. Substitution on this amino acid by another positive-charged residue has only small effects on ATP sensitivity whereas the substitution with a neutral or negative-charged amino acid causes major impairment in channel function [14, 52–54]. However, the decrease in ATP sensitivity due to R201 mutation remains small and therefore is responsible for isolated neonatal diabetes whereas those causing greater reduction like V59M, V59G, Q52R are associated with severe disease [14, 47, 48, 51]. The first 4 mutations identified [49, 55] in transient neonatal diabetes (R201H, G53S, G53R and I182V) result in milder reductions in ATP sensitivity but the phenotype associated is variable as the mothers of the probands had permanent neonatal diabetes or diabetes developing after 5 years of age in 3 out of 4 cases. The muscle weakness observed can have both a muscular and neurological basis as Kir6.2 is expressed in both cells. The developmental delay and epilepsy result from defective K_{ATP} channels present in the central nervous system as described earlier. Conversely, no marked effect has been described on the heart function or the ECG, which may be explained by the greater ATP inhibition of mutant Kir6.2/SUR2A than of Kir6.2/SUR1 [51, 56, 57].

As explained, the K_{ATP} channel, composed of SUR1 and Kir6.2 proteins, is a key regulator of insulin release. It is inhibited by the binding of adenine nucleotides to Kir6.2, which closes the channel, and is activated by nucleotide binding and/or hydrolysis on SUR1, which opens the channel. The balance of these opposing actions determines the low open-channel probability, which controls the excitability of pancreatic β-cells. We hypothesized that activating mutations in *ABCC8*, which encodes SUR1, cause neonatal diabetes. We therefore screened the 39 exons of *ABCC8* in 34 patients diagnosed with permanent or transient neonatal diabetes of unknown origin in a case series of 73 patients with neonatal diabetes [58]. We assayed the electrophysiological activity of mutant and wild-type K_{ATP} channels. We identified 7 missense mutations in 9 patients. Four mutations were familial and showed vertical transmission with neonatal and adult-onset diabetes; the remaining mutations were de novo and not found in more than 300 nondiabetic or early-onset diabetic subjects of similar genetic background. Mutant channels in intact cells and in physiologic concentrations of MgATP had a markedly higher open-channel probability compared with wild-type channels. These overactive channels retained sulphonylurea sensitivity and treatment with sulphonylureas achieved euglycemia. Dominant mutations in *ABCC8* account for 12% (9/73) of our neonatal diabetes cases. Diabetes results from a novel mechanism whereby the basal Mg-nucleotide-dependent stimulatory action of SUR1 on the Kir pore is elevated and block by sulphonylureas is preserved [58]. Further cases with SUR1 mutations are being described [59–61]. In the French network, most of the mutations in SUR1 were associated with transient neonatal diabetes mellitus whereas Kir6.2 mutations were associated with early-onset (before 6 months) permanent neonatal diabetes mellitus [61]. The phenotypic variability of SUR1 mutations is broader [58]. Indeed mutations in SUR1 can be linked to ketoacidosis in a newborn as well as to bona fide type 2 diabetes in a young adult [58, and its supplementary web information].

In the English case series with transient neonatal diabetes mellitus, mutations in SUR1 explained as many cases as mutations in Kir6.2 [60]. This discrepancy deserves further exploration.

Therapeutic Consequences: Use of Sulphonylurea in Adults and Children with ATP-Sensitive Potassium Channel Gene Mutations

The sulphonylurea effect on pancreatic β-cells was discovered in 1942 by Janbon as patients treated for typhoid fever developed severe hypoglycemia. Thereafter, the sulphonylurea family developed rapidly and has been used as treatment for diabetes not requiring insulin since 1956 [62]. Sulphonylureas close K_{ATP} channels by binding with high affinity to SUR [57, 63, 64]. In the absence of added nucleotides, high-affinity inhibition of the K_{ATP} current by sulphonylurea reaches only 60–80% [17].

SUR1 possesses two binding sites for glibenclamide whereas tolbutamide binds only to one [2, 57, 62]. This double binding may explain the glibenclamide long washout time [65]. Besides binding the pancreatic K_{ATP} channel, glibenclamide inhibits the activity of cardiac and skeletal or smooth muscle type channel [65] but also mi-

Table 1. Case reports of successful transfer from insulin to sulfonylurea oral therapy for patients with a *KCNJ11* mutation

Reference	Age at diabetes	Age at time of transfer	Kir6.2 mutation	Glibenclamide
Gloyn et al. [14] (1 patient)	<3 years	46 years	R201H	tolbutamide since childhood
Sagen et al. [68] (3 patients)	10 months	2 years	F333I	0.4 mg/kg/day stop insulin in 62 days
	2 weeks	6 years	R201H	0.4 mg/kg/day stop insulin in 2 weeks
	1 week	1 year	V59M	0.3 mg/kg/day stop insulin in 8 weeks
Zung et al. [66] (1 patient)	68 years	9.5 months	R201H	0.8 mg/kg/day stop insulin in 3 days
Codner et al. [67] (1 patient)	4 months	17 months	R201L	0.8 mg/kg/day stop insulin in 8 weeks
Klupa et al. [69] (1 patient)	3 months	9.5 years	R201H	0.18 mg/kg/day stop insulin in 5 days
Pearson et al. [70] (49 patients)	0.5–3 months	3 months to 36 years	F35V, H46Y, G53N, G53R, V59M (n = 6), K170T, R201C (n = 5), R201H (n = 23), R201L, E322K, Y330S, F333I	successful transfer (n = 44) 0.45 mg/kg/day (0.05–1.5)
			Q52R, G53R, L164P, R201C, I296L	unsuccessful from insulin to sulfonylurea

tochondrial channels by binding to SUR2. Yet, this affinity of glibenclamide for SUR2 is 300- to 500-fold lower than for SUR1. Nevertheless, precautions may have to be taken when treating patients with ischemic heart disease at a high dose of glibenclamide [65] as the K_{ATP} channels intervene in the cardioprotective mechanism of ischemia-related preconditioning as described above. However, the absence of side effects of this type reported in type 2 diabetes treatment suggests that the effects of extra pancreatic channel inhibition might be subtle.

The high affinity of sulphonylurea for the pancreatic K_{ATP} channels suggested that these drugs may be used to replace insulin in these patients. Intravenous injection of tolbutamide could stimulate insulin secretion in patients with a *KCNJ11* mutation even when they did not respond to intravenous glucose [14]. Subsequently, 7 patients had been successfully switched from subcutaneous insulin injections to oral sulphonylurea therapy [14, 66–69] (table 1). The dose of glibenclamide required has been up to 0.8 mg/kg/day, which is a much higher dose than that used for type 2 diabetes treatment. The delay needed to stop insulin is between 3 days and 8 weeks with a follow-up of nearly 2 years now. These results show great heterogeneity between the patients, even with the same *KCNJ11* mutations. Our own experience shows a successful transfer from insulin to oral glibenclamide for 4 patients out of 6, the last 2 girls unable to transfer being twins with neurological features probably related to another pathology not yet understood, and for whom compliance was probably suboptimal.

Our recent European collaborative study reported a total of 49 consecutive patients (from 3 months to 36 years old) from 40 families having permanent neonatal diabetes due to heterozygous mutation of *KCNJ11* [70]. Of these 49 patients treated with an adequate dose of sulphonylureas (0.8 mg/kg/day equivalent glibenclamide), 44 (90%) were able to stop insulin treatment. The median dose of glibenclamide initially required was 0.45 mg/kg/day (0.05–1.5 mg/kg/day). Glycemic control improved in all 38 patients tested with a mean glycated hemoglobin level falling from 8.1% before sulphonylurea to 6.4% at 12 weeks after cessation of insulin, without enhancing the frequency of hypoglycemia. Eighty percent (4 out of 5) of the patients unable to stop insulin had neurologic features in contrast with only 14% (6 out of 44) in the successful group. Five patients had transitory diarrhea; no other side effect was reported. Some studies have shown that closure of K_{ATP} channels by sulphonylurea therapy could induce β-cell apoptosis in human islets and therefore precipitate the decrease in the β-cell mass in type 2 diabetes patients, but this needs further clarification [71, 72]. However, in consideration of patients, with *KCNJ11* mutations, even if glibenclamide efficacy is transitory lasting for several years, it means years without daily subcutaneous injections and the subsequent improvement of quality of life.

Transfer from Insulin to Glibenclamide: A Case Study

We designed a protocol to transfer children with insulin-treated diabetes due to *KCNJ11* and *ABCC8* mutations from insulin to sulphonylurea and evaluate them, as the use of this drug is not allowed for children in our country, France. We got the approval of the Clinical Research Direction of our institution (AP-HP, Paris, France), as well as the agreement of the ethics committee and of the French Authorities for Health Care (AFSSAPS), to include the children identified so far with such diabetes.

We here report the case of a 37-year-old patient with permanent neonatal diabetes discovered at the age of 2 months during a systematic glucose monitoring as she was hospitalized for bilateral otitis. Metabolic control was fair under appropriate diet until she was 5 years when insulin therapy was initiated. However, despite several times when injections were withdrawn for several days, she never had ketoacidosis. She had 2 children, the first one being a girl who developed permanent neonatal diabetes on the first day of life and was immediately treated with insulin injections. The Kir6.2 mutation R201H was found in 2004 for both mother and daughter and we started glibenclamide therapy in January 2005. The transfer was a great success as the first

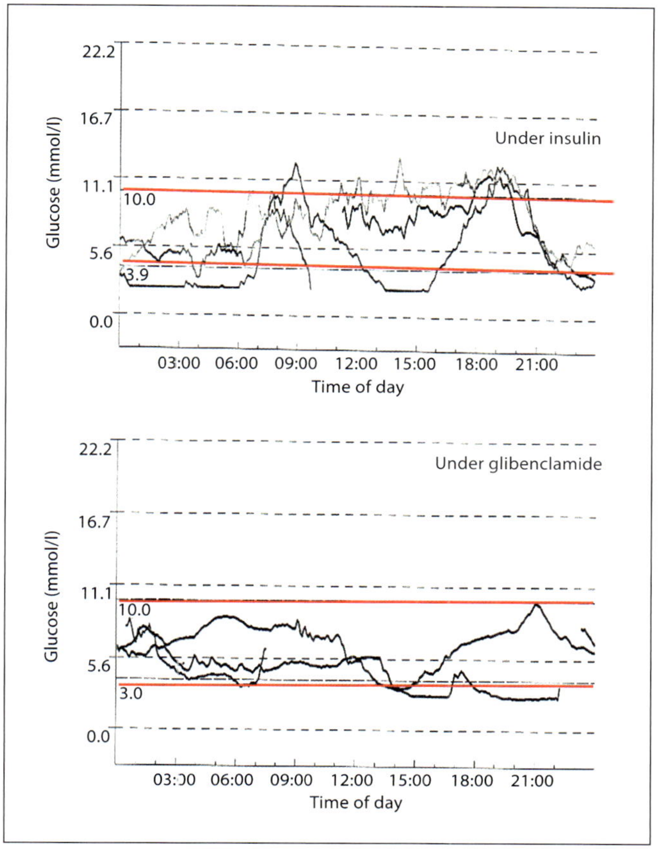

Fig. 4. Continuous monitoring of glycemia during 3 days of a 37-year-old patient with R201H mutation, first under insulin and then under glibenclamide. See the decrease in the variability of the glycemic level after the transfer to glibenclamide.

tablet taken was sufficient to permanently negate the requirement for insulin injections for both, with a required dose under 0.1 mg/kg/day of glibenclamide (mother at 36 years of age, daughter at 15 years of age). They both improved their glycemic control and their HbA1c level (from 7.4 to 6% for the mother and from 9.5 to 7.9% for the daughter) with more than 2 years of follow-up and no side effects, particularly no recurrent hypoglycemia. As shown in figure 4, the glycemic values were much steadier under glibenclamide than under insulin therapy.

In conclusion, the K_{ATP} channels play a central role in cellular response to metabolic changes in many organs and especially in the pancreatic β-cells. Advances in the comprehension of the physiological function of these channels have identified a major clinical application for patients having permanent neonatal diabetes due to mutations in the *KCNJ11* or *ABCC8* genes. The transfer from insulin injections to oral glibenclamide therapy seems highly effective and safe for most patients [58, 59, 61,

66–70]. It illustrates how the molecular understanding of some monogenic forms of diabetes has led to an unexpected, but highly effective change of the treatment in children. This is a spectacular example by which a pharmacogenomic approach tremendously improves way the quality of life of our young patients.

Acknowledgments

We would like to thank for their participation in the studies of the French study group of neonatal diabetes: Drs. and Profs. Badet-Marti in Palamos, Spain; Bertrand in Besançon, Tubiana and Robert in Paris, Crosnier in Saint Germain-en-Laye, Doremus in Cambrai, Garandeau in Palavas-les-Flots, all in France; Khallouf in Beyrouth, Lebanon; Loeuille in Dunkerque, Nivot-Adamiak in Rennes, France; Phillip and Nimri in Petah Tikva, Israel; Pradines in Grenoble, Stuckens in Lille, France; Dundar in Turkey; Fernandez and Fernandez-Rebollo in Bilbao, Spain; Gonthier in Montréal, Canada; Lechuga in Cadiz, Spain; Metz and Giroux in Brest, Soskin in Strasbourg, Sulmont in Reims, France; Perez de Nanclares and Luis Castaño in Barakaldo, Spain. We would like to thank all of the families for their participation in the study. We are very grateful to Prof. Paul Czernichow for his continuous support of the projects dedicated to neonatal diabetes, and to Dr. Lydia Aguilar-Bryan for her helpful discussions. Our studies were supported by the European Union (Integrated Project EuroDia LSHM-CT-2006-518153 in the Framework Program 6 of the European Community; to M.V. and P.F.). We also acknowledge the French nonprofit associations Aide aux Jeunes Diabétiques (to M.P.) and Association Française des Diabétiques (to R.S.) for their support of parts of the study.

References

1 Bryan J, et al: Insulin secretagogues, sulfonylurea receptors and K(ATP) channels. Curr Pharm Des 2005;11:2699–2716.

2 Mikhailov MV, et al: 3-D structural and functional characterization of the purified K_{ATP} channel complex Kir6.2-SUR1. EMBO J 2005;24:4166–4175.

3 Bond CT, et al: Cloning and functional expression of the cDNA encoding an inwardly-rectifying potassium channel expressed in pancreatic beta-cells and in the brain. FEBS Lett 1995;367:61–66.

4 Clement JPT, et al: Association and stoichiometry of K(ATP) channel subunits. Neuron 1997;18:827–838.

5 Inagaki N, et al: A family of sulfonylurea receptors determines the pharmacological properties of ATP-sensitive K^+ channels. Neuron 1996;16:1011–1017.

6 Isomoto S, et al: A novel sulfonylurea receptor forms with BIR (Kir6.2) a smooth muscle type ATP-sensitive K^+ channel. J Biol Chem 1996;271: 24321–24324.

7 Inagaki N, et al: Reconstitution of IK_{ATP}: an inward rectifier subunit plus the sulfonylurea receptor. Science 1995;270:1166–1170.

8 Gopel SO, et al: Regulation of glucagon release in mouse-cells by K_{ATP} channels and inactivation of TTX-sensitive Na^+ channels. J Physiol 2000;528: 509–520.

9 Gopel SO, et al: Patch-clamp characterisation of somatostatin-secreting cells in intact mouse pancreatic islets. J Physiol 2000;528:497–507.

10 Gribble FM, et al: A novel glucose-sensing mechanism contributing to glucagon-like peptide-1 secretion from the GLUTag cell line. Diabetes 2003;52: 1147–1154.

11 Cook DL, et al: ATP-sensitive K^+ channels in pancreatic beta-cells. Spare-channel hypothesis. Diabetes 1988;37:495–498.

12 Aguilar-Bryan L, et al: Cloning of the beta cell high-affinity sulfonylurea receptor: a regulator of insulin secretion. Science 1995;268:423–426.

13 Gribble FM, et al: Properties of cloned ATP-sensitive K^+ currents expressed in Xenopus oocytes. J Physiol 1997;498:87–98.

14 Gloyn AL, et al: Activating mutations in the gene encoding the ATP-sensitive potassium-channel subunit Kir6.2 and permanent neonatal diabetes. N Engl J Med 2004;350:1838–1849.

15 Winarto A, et al: Morphological changes in pancreatic islets of K_{ATP} channel-deficient mice: the involvement of K_{ATP} channels in the survival of insulin cells and the maintenance of islet architecture. Arch Histol Cytol 2001;64:59–67.
16 Miki T, et al: Roles of ATP-sensitive K^+ channels in cell survival and differentiation in the endocrine pancreas. Diabetes 2001;50(suppl 1):S48–S51.
17 Proks P, et al: Sulfonylurea stimulation of insulin secretion. Diabetes 2002;51(suppl 3):S368–S376.
18 Seino S, Miki T: Gene targeting approach to clarification of ion channel function: studies of Kir6.x null mice. J Physiol 2004;554:295–300.
19 Dunn-Meynell AA, Rawson NE, Levin BE: Distribution and phenotype of neurons containing the ATP-sensitive K^+ channel in rat brain. Brain Res 1998;814:41–54.
20 Yamada K, Inagaki N: Neuroprotection by K_{ATP} channels. J Mol Cell Cardiol 2005;38:945–949.
21 Heron-Milhavet L, et al: Protection against hypoxic-ischemic injury in transgenic mice overexpressing Kir6.2 channel pore in forebrain. Mol Cell Neurosci 2004;54:585–593.
22 Yamada K, Inagaki N: ATP-sensitive K(+) channels in the brain: sensors of hypoxic conditions. News Physiol Sci 2002;17:127–130.
23 Miki T, et al: ATP-sensitive K^+ channels in the hypothalamus are essential for the maintenance of glucose homeostasis. Nat Neurosci 2001;4:507–512.
24 Deacon RM, et al: Behavioral phenotyping of mice lacking the K_{ATP} channel subunit Kir6.2. Physiol Behav 2006;87:723–733.
25 Gong B, et al: K_{ATP} channels depress force by reducing action potential amplitude in mouse EDL and soleus muscle. Am J Physiol Cell Physiol 2003;285: C1464–C1474.
26 Zingman LV, et al: Kir6.2 is required for adaptation to stress. Proc Natl Acad Sci USA 2002;99:13278–13283.
27 Hodgson DM, et al: Cellular remodeling in heart failure disrupts K(ATP) channel-dependent stress tolerance. EMBO J 2003;22:1732–1742.
28 Kane GC, et al: ATP-sensitive K^+ channel knockout compromises the metabolic benefit of exercise training, resulting in cardiac deficits. Diabetes 2004;53(suppl 3):S169–S175.
29 Terzic A, Jahangir A, Kurachi Y: Cardiac ATP-sensitive K^+ channels: regulation by intracellular nucleotides and K^+ channel-opening drugs. Am J Physiol 1995;269:C525–C545.
30 Nichols CG, Lederer WJ: Adenosine triphosphate-sensitive potassium channels in the cardiovascular system. Am J Physiol 1991;261:H1675–H1686.
31 Liu XK, et al: Genetic disruption of Kir6.2, the pore-forming subunit of ATP-sensitive K^+ channel, predisposes to catecholamine-induced ventricular dysrhythmia. Diabetes 2004;53(suppl 3):S165–S168.
32 Suzuki M, et al: Role of sarcolemmal K(ATP) channels in cardioprotection against ischemia/reperfusion injury in mice. J Clin Invest 2002;109:509–516.
33 Bienengraeber M, et al: ABCC9 mutations identified in human dilated cardiomyopathy disrupt catalytic K_{ATP} channel gating. Nat Genet 2004;36:382–387.
34 Quayle JM, Nelson MT, Standen NB: ATP-sensitive and inwardly rectifying potassium channels in smooth muscle. Physiol Rev 1997;77:1165–1232.
35 Kleppisch T, Nelson MT: ATP-sensitive K^+ currents in cerebral arterial smooth muscle: pharmacological and hormonal modulation. Am J Physiol 1995; 269:H1634–H1640.
36 Iafusco D, et al: Permanent diabetes mellitus in the first year of life. Diabetologia 2002;45:798–804.
37 Koster JC, et al: Targeted overactivity of beta cell K(ATP) channels induces profound neonatal diabetes. Cell 2000;100:645–654.
38 Hani EH, et al: A missense mutation in hepatocyte nuclear factor-4 alpha, resulting in a reduced transactivation activity, in human late-onset non-insulin-dependent diabetes mellitus. J Clin Invest 1998; 101:521–526.
39 Gloyn AL, et al: Large-scale association studies of variants in genes encoding the pancreatic beta-cell K_{ATP} channel subunits Kir6.2 (KCNJ11) and SUR1 (ABCC8) confirm that the KCNJ11 E23K variant is associated with type 2 diabetes. Diabetes 2003;52: 568–572.
40 Florez JC, et al: Haplotype structure and genotype-phenotype correlations of the sulfonylurea receptor and the islet ATP-sensitive potassium channel gene region. Diabetes 2004;53:1360–1368.
41 Tschritter O, et al: The prevalent Glu23Lys polymorphism in the potassium inward rectifier 6.2 (KIR6.2) gene is associated with impaired glucagon suppression in response to hyperglycemia. Diabetes 2002;51:2854–2860.
42 Polak M, Shield J: Neonatal and very-early-onset diabetes mellitus. Semin Neonatol 2004;9:59–65.
43 Metz C, et al: Neonatal diabetes mellitus: chromosomal analysis in transient and permanent cases. J Pediatr 2002;141:483–489.
44 Njolstad PR, et al: Neonatal diabetes mellitus due to complete glucokinase deficiency. N Engl J Med 2001;344:1588–1592.
45 Njolstad PR, et al: Permanent neonatal diabetes caused by glucokinase deficiency: inborn error of the glucose-insulin signaling pathway. Diabetes 2003;52:2854–2860.
46 Edghill EL, et al: Activating mutations in the KCNJ11 gene encoding the ATP-sensitive K^+ channel subunit Kir6.2 are rare in clinically defined type 1 diabetes diagnosed before 2 years. Diabetes 2004; 53:2998–3001.

47 Vaxillaire M, et al: Kir6.2 mutations are a common cause of permanent neonatal diabetes in a large cohort of French patients. Diabetes 2004;53:2719–2722.
48 Massa O, et al: KCNJ11 activating mutations in Italian patients with permanent neonatal diabetes. Hum Mutat 2005;25:22–27.
49 Gloyn AL, et al: Relapsing diabetes can result from moderately activating mutations in KCNJ11. Hum Mol Genet 2005;14:925–934.
50 Gloyn AL, et al: Permanent neonatal diabetes due to paternal germline mosaicism for an activating mutation of the KCNJ11 gene encoding the Kir6.2 subunit of the beta-cell potassium adenosine triphosphate channel. J Clin Endocrinol Metab 2004; 89:3932–3935.
51 Proks P, et al: Molecular basis of Kir6.2 mutations associated with neonatal diabetes or neonatal diabetes plus neurological features. Proc Natl Acad Sci USA 2004;101:17539–17544.
52 Antcliff JF, et al: Functional analysis of a structural model of the ATP-binding site of the K_{ATP} channel Kir6.2 subunit. EMBO J 2005;24:229–239.
53 John SA, et al: Molecular mechanism for ATP-dependent closure of the K^+ channel Kir6.2. J Physiol 2003;552:23–34.
54 Ribalet B, John SA, Weiss JN: Molecular basis for Kir6.2 channel inhibition by adenine nucleotides. Biophys J 2003;84:266–276.
55 Colombo C, et al: Transient neonatal diabetes mellitus is associated with a recurrent (R201H) KCNJ11 (KIR6.2) mutation. Diabetologia 2005;48:2439–2441.
56 Tammaro P, Proks P, Ashcroft FM: Functional effects of naturally occurring KCNJ11 mutations causing neonatal diabetes on cloned cardiac K_{ATP} channels. J Physiol 2006;571:3–14.
57 Gribble FM, et al: Tissue specificity of sulfonylureas: studies on cloned cardiac and beta-cell K(ATP) channels. Diabetes 1998;47:1412–1418.
58 Babenko AP, et al: Activating mutations in the ABCC8 gene in neonatal diabetes mellitus. N Engl J Med 2006;355:456–466.
59 Stanik J, et al: Prevalence of permanent neonatal diabetes in Slovakia and successful replacement of insulin with sulfonylurea therapy in KCNJ11 and ABCC8 mutation carriers. J Clin Endocrinol Metab 2007;92:1276–1282.
60 Flanagan SE, et al: Mutations in K_{ATP} channel genes cause transient neonatal diabetes and permanent diabetes in childhood and adulthood. Diabetes 2007;56:1930–1937.
61 Vaxillaire M, et al: New ABCC8 mutations in relapsing neonatal diabetes and clinical features. Diabetes 2007;56:1737–1741.
62 Henquin JC: Pathways in beta-cell stimulus-secretion coupling as targets for therapeutic insulin secretagogues. Diabetes 2004;53(suppl 3):S48–S58.
63 Gribble FM, Ashcroft FM: Differential sensitivity of beta-cell and extrapancreatic K(ATP) channels to gliclazide. Diabetologia 1999;42:845–848.
64 Gribble FM, Tucker SJ, Ashcroft FM: The interaction of nucleotides with the tolbutamide block of cloned ATP-sensitive K^+ channel currents expressed in Xenopus oocytes: a reinterpretation. J Physiol 1997;504:35–45.
65 Nagashima K, et al: Sulfonylurea and non-sulfonylurea hypoglycemic agents: pharmachological properties and tissue selectivity. Diabetes Res Clin Pract 2004;66(suppl 1):S75–S78.
66 Zung A, et al: Glibenclamide treatment in permanent neonatal diabetes mellitus due to an activating mutation in Kir6.2. J Clin Endocrinol Metab 2004; 89:5504–5507.
67 Codner E, et al: High-dose glibenclamide can replace insulin therapy despite transitory diarrhea in early-onset diabetes caused by a novel R201L Kir6.2 mutation. Diabetes Care 2005;28:758–759.
68 Sagen JV, et al: Permanent neonatal diabetes due to mutations in KCNJ11 encoding Kir6.2: patient characteristics and initial response to sulfonylurea therapy. Diabetes 2004;53:2713–2718.
69 Klupa T, et al: The identification of a R201H mutation in KCNJ11, which encodes Kir6.2, and successful transfer to sustained-release sulphonylurea therapy in a subject with neonatal diabetes: evidence for heterogeneity of beta cell function among carriers of the R201H mutation. Diabetologia 2005; 48:1029–1031.
70 Pearson ER, et al: Switching from insulin to oral sulfonylureas in patients with diabetes due to Kir6.2 mutations. N Engl J Med 2006;355:467–477.
71 Maedler K, et al: Sulfonylurea induced beta-cell apoptosis in cultured human islets. J Clin Endocrinol Metab 2005;90:501–506.
72 Rustenbeck I, et al: Beta-cell toxicity of ATP-sensitive K^+ channel-blocking insulin secretagogues. Biochem Pharmacol 2004;67:1733–1741.

Dr. Michel Polak
Clinique des Maladies du Développement, Unité d'Endocrinologie
Diabétologie et Gynécologie Pédiatrique, Hôpital Necker-Enfants Malades
149, rue de Sèvres, FR–75015 Paris (France)
Tel. +33 1 4449 4802, Fax +33 1 4438 1648, E-Mail michel.polak@nck.aphp.fr

Shield JPH, Scharfmann R (eds): Development of the Pancreas and Neonatal Diabetes.
Endocr Dev. Basel, Karger, 2007, vol 12, pp 99–112

Genomic Imprinting – Roles and Regulation in Development

Gavin Kelsey

Laboratory of Developmental Genetics and Imprinting, The Babraham Institute, Cambridge, UK

Abstract

Genomic imprinting results in the deliberate silencing of alleles, dictated by their parental origin, but reversible on passage through the germ line. In this chapter, we shall consider the functional properties of imprinted genes, why these genes might have been singled out for the risky strategy of mono-allelic expression, and how imprinting is regulated. We shall look at how imprinted genes affect processes throughout our lifetimes, from the way we grow in the womb to the control of metabolism as adults. In contrast to the depth of our knowledge of the contributions of imprinted genes to growth of the fetus, our understanding of their roles in adult physiology is still rather poor. We shall look at those imprinted genes that have been implicated in diabetes and those which are known to help determine β-cell mass. It is likely that the effects of imprinted genes on these processes are more pervasive than currently recognised. The intention of this chapter is therefore to equip the readers with the general principles governing imprinting, so that they are able to comprehend this intriguing and important form of gene regulation when they encounter it next.

What Is Imprinting?

Genomic imprinting is a special form of gene regulation in mammals that results in the silencing of one copy, or allele, of a given gene [1]. This 'mono-allelic' silencing affects only a subset of autosomal genes and is strictly determined by parental origin, meaning that there are imprinted genes for which the maternally derived allele is always silenced and imprinted genes for which the paternally derived allele is always silent. Imprinting occurs because these genes receive specific marks, referred to as imprints, during development of the male and female germ cells. These imprints are faithfully maintained after fertilisation, and at every successive cell division, such that the two alleles have a permanent memory of the parent from which they derived.

These marks then determine whether the allele is active or silent in the somatic tissues of the individual. Thus, imprinting represents a unique state in that active and silent copies of the same gene coexist in the same nucleus. Importantly, however, the process is reversible, such that the marks are erased and reset in the germ line. These characteristics of modification of gene function independent of sequence changes but with parental legacy qualify imprinting as an epigenetic mechanism.

As a phenomenon in mammals, imprinting was recognised a little over 20 years ago and the first imprinted genes were identified in 1991 [2]. Our insights into the functions of imprinting, the reasons for its existence, how it is regulated and the pathological consequences when imprinting is disrupted come from studies of human disorders and from the mouse as a model organism. Since the early 1990s, there has been an explosion of interest and understanding of this intriguing phenomenon. We now know of the existence of about 80 imprinted genes in the mouse and human genomes [3]. Although this represents a small proportion of our total gene content, at a functional level imprinted genes are very important in mammalian development and physiology, and may be involved in more than their fair share of genetic disorders [4]. Imprinted genes are rather unevenly distributed across the genome and many imprinted genes exist in large clusters [1]. This is important, as it suggests that single *cis*-acting regulatory elements, known as imprinting control regions (ICRs), within each cluster may be responsible for imprinting of multiple genes. There is generally good concordance in the genes that are imprinted in humans and in other mammals, where it is known (e.g. mice), although there are exceptions [3]. Certainly, the major imprinted clusters appear generally to be conserved. This suggests that these genes are under strong selective pressure to be imprinted. Genomic imprinting is known to exist in eutherian mammals and a few genes have also been found to be similarly imprinted in marsupials [5]. This form of imprinting is not thought to exist in vertebrates outside of the mammalian lineage.

Why Is Imprinting Important?

Imprinting poses a number of problems. The fact that one potentially functional allele has been deliberately silenced denies that gene any backup against mutation arising in the single active copy. A disease resulting from mutation in an imprinted gene will therefore present an autosomal dominant mode of inheritance, but with sex-limited transmission. This can be seen in a number of diseases with an imprinted aetiology. Inactivating mutations in the cyclin-dependent kinase p57Kip2 (*CDKN1C* gene) have been found as one cause for the imprinted growth and development disorder Beckwith-Wiedemann syndrome when the mutations are transmitted maternally [6]. Similarly, Angelman syndrome (AS), which results in severe mental retardation, can be caused by inactivating mutations in the imprinted gene *UBE3A,* again only on maternal transmission [7, 8].

The flip side is that if mammals have chosen deliberately to silence one allele of a functionally important gene, there may be consequences of having both copies active, which is referred to as loss of imprinting (LoI). This occurs, for example, in transient neonatal diabetes mellitus (TNDM) with a 6q24 aetiology [see chapter by I. Karen Temple, this vol., pp. 113–123]. TNDM presents as severe intra-uterine growth restriction (IUGR), hyperglycaemia and absence of detectable insulin in the perinatal period, sometimes with additional manifestations, such as macroglossia [9]. The basis of the disease is not fully understood, but presumably reflects an acute failure of β-cells to produce or secrete insulin during the final trimester. Through a variety of genetic analyses, a critical interval for TNDM has been defined, and a number of genetic causes of TNDM identified, including paternal uniparental isodisomy for chromosome 6 and paternally derived duplications of 6q24 [9]. In addition, an epigenetic anomaly – loss of methylation of the candidate gene – has been found [10, 11]. All point to a similar possible underlying cause, i.e., two-fold overexpression of the single candidate imprinted locus, *PLAGL1/ZAC1*. This illustrates that a simple increase in expression of a single imprinted locus can have profound consequences on endocrine pancreas development and/or function.

Because imprinting relies on epigenetic mechanisms, there is a potential for such mechanisms to be vulnerable to deregulation, resulting in aberrant imprinted gene expression. The assumption is that once an imprint mark is lost in some way, it cannot be restored in somatic tissues and will only be reset on subsequent passage through the germ line [12]. Therefore, early events which disrupt an imprint will have lifelong consequences for the expression of the gene(s) affected. There are a number of conditions in which this appears to occur. For example, an increased incidence of imprinted gene syndromes has been described associated with assisted reproductive techniques such as in vitro fertilisation and intracytoplasmic sperm injection [13]. This notion also lies behind the current speculation that imprinted genes may be involved in developmental programming events, wherein suboptimal conditions during pregnancy, resulting for example in IUGR, can result in an enhanced risk for chronic diseases of adulthood, such as type 2 diabetes and hypertension, or the so-called metabolic syndrome [14, 15].

Aberrant imprinting also occurs in cancer. LoI for *IGF2* (and the neighbouring *H19* gene) was first identified in the paediatric Wilms' tumour [16, 17]. It is thought that the predicted overexpression of this important mitogen provides a growth advantage to transformed cells, and LoI for *IGF2* has subsequently been described in a great variety of tumours [18]. A number of other imprinted genes have also been implicated in cancer [18]. For an imprinted gene with a potential role as a tumour suppressor, such as *PLAGL1/ZAC1* [19], the normal mono-allelic silencing thus requires only a single 'hit' in the active allele to completely eliminate tumour suppressor function.

Why Do We Have Imprinting?

In view of these problems associated with imprinting and its potential for deregulation, it might legitimately be asked: 'why do we bother to have imprinting?' There must be a significant selective advantage in the mono-allelic silencing of these genes, especially given the general conservation of imprinting between humans and mice, to offset against these potentially deleterious consequences. The answer can be found, fortuitously, in the very first imprinted genes to have been discovered in mice: they do seem to provide us with some of the overriding principles for imprinting, as was recognised at the time by Haig and Graham [20]. The first known imprinted genes were *Igf2,* which encodes the key fetal mitogen, insulin-like growth factor 2; *Igf2r,* encoding the type 2 IGF receptor, and the non-coding RNA *H19.* Knockouts in mice reveal that each of these genes has a profound effect on growth of the fetus. Thus, inactivation of the single active copy of *Igf2* results in mice with an approximately 40% reduction in birth weight [21], whereas mutations resulting in LoI of *Igf2,* such that both copies of the gene are active, enhance birth weight by about 30% [22]. Conversely, inactivating mutations of *Igf2r* enhance weight at term by about 30% [23]; LoI of *Igf2r* leading to overexpression reduces pup weight by approximately 20% [24]. These effects can be explained because a major function of the type 2 IGF receptor in mammals is to sequester circulating IGF2 for degradation in lysosomes. Similarly, deletion of the *H19* gene causes enhanced term weight and *H19* LoI reduces term weight [22, 25]. Again, these outcomes can be explained by an effect on *Igf2* levels, because the only accepted function of the *H19* gene is to regulate the imprinting of *Igf2*. *Igf2* is imprinted such that the maternal allele is silenced, whereas for *Igf2r* and *H19* the paternal allele is silenced. These observations illustrate, first, that three imprinted genes operate towards a single outcome, i.e., to control the size of the fetus and, second, that paternally expressed imprinted genes and maternally expressed imprinted genes function antagonistically in this common pathway. This appears to be a fundamental principle in genomic imprinting that the reader is encouraged to note.

If we look at the phenotypes resulting from knockouts of imprinted genes that have been done over the past two decades, it is striking that effects on fetal growth predominate (table 1). Furthermore, the trend for paternally expressed genes to promote birth weight and for maternally expressed genes to restrict fetal or placental weight is obvious. These genes encode a variety of different functions, including putative transcription factors, growth factors and their receptors, signalling proteins; for some the function is not fully clear. Despite this diversity of molecular, biochemical or cellular functions, they are united in having a significant effect on controlling the growth of the fetus.

With these observations in mind, it is now possible to consider why imprinting exists. The discovery of the imprinting of *Igf2* and *Igf2r* provided early support to a theory for the evolution of imprinting in mammals that has become known as the 'conflict hypothesis', which arises out of the kinship theory [26]. Put briefly, paternal

Table 1. Imprinted genes affecting fetal and placental growth in mice

Gene	Expressed allele	Null phenotype		Reference
		weight at term[1]	placenta[1]	
Ascl1	maternal	lethality	spongiotrophoblast failure	68
Cdkn1c	maternal	lethality	increased growth	69
Dlk1	paternal	reduced	not known	70
Grb10	maternal	increased	increased growth	71
H19	maternal	increased	increased growth	22
Igf2	paternal	reduced	reduced growth	21
Igf2r	maternal	increased	increased growth	23
Mest	paternal	reduced	reduced growth	72
Peg3	paternal	reduced	reduced growth	73
Phlda2	maternal	normal	increased growth	74
Zac1	paternal	reduced	normal	75

[1] Describes the effect of targeted disruption of the gene. Most effects relate to mice heterozygous for inactivating mutations, where the mutations are carried on the normally active allele. Homozygous mutants are expected to be similarly affected.

alleles in offspring cannot predict their relatedness to future paternal alleles in offspring from the same mother, whereas maternal alleles in offspring will be equally related in all offspring from a given female irrespective of offspring paternity. This sets up a tension between paternal and maternal genes, such that paternal genes seek to extract more resources from the mother than her optimum to provide, at a potential cost to the future reproductive output of the mother (in which the paternal genes may have no relatives). Maternal genes in offspring have an additional interest in conserving maternal resources for the future reproductive output of that mother. This tension arises particularly in placental mammals, because the fetus (and its paternal genes) has the opportunity to manipulate the resources it acquires from the mother during growth and development in utero in a way that is not possible in egg-laying mammals and other vertebrates, because of the extensive maternal postfertilisation provisioning. By this logic, it is also to be expected that imprinted genes may control resource acquisition and utilisation by offspring in the postnatal preweaning period when the infant remains fully dependent on the mother for food through suckling [4, 26]. In this context, imprinted genes have been found whose major action is after birth during the critical neonatal period [27].

This theory for the evolution of imprinting has become quite widely accepted and appears to be the best of the current ones in explaining the available observations, in particular the phylogenetic distribution of imprinting and direction of parental allele effects [28], and provides a very useful general principle for understanding and predicting quite diverse physiological effects of imprinted genes. For example, Haig and Wharton [29] have suggested a 'conflict' explanation for the neonatal feeding difficulties but subsequent insatiable appetite and morbid obesity of Prader-Willi syndrome patients; others have attempted the same for the characteristic happy demeanour and soliciting behaviour of AS children [30]. However, some effects of imprinted genes appear to be at odds with the predictions of the kinship theory and it is not without its critics [31].

How Is Imprinting Regulated?

The imprinting life cycle comprises phases of establishment, maintenance and resetting, as well as translation of imprint marks into differential gene expression [1]. As stated earlier, imprinting arises because of distinct 'epigenetic marks' applied to these genes in germ cells. A major component of the imprint mark is DNA methylation, wherein an ICR becomes densely methylated in one germ line but not the other. Most imprint marks correspond to DNA methylation laid down in the female germ line, during the growth phase of the oocyte [32]; only 3 imprint marks are known to arise in the male germ line. Germ line imprint establishment involves the de novo methyltransferase Dnmt3a [33], and the related protein Dnmt3l, certainly in oocytes [34, 35]. What singles out these regions for acquisition of imprint marks is not clear, although factors such as repeated sequence motifs and intronic location have been discussed [36, 37]. Imprint marks then have to survive periods of extensive epigenetic reprogramming of the genome during pre-implantation and post-implantation development [38], as these marks normally accompany the parental alleles throughout the lifetime of the organism.

DNA methylation, either directly or acting in concert with histone modifications and other chromosomal proteins [39], has the capacity to determine gene activity of imprinted genes in a number of ways (fig. 1). The most direct occurs where the DNA methylation mark sits on the promoter of an imprinted gene, leading to silencing of that allele. This occurs, for example, in the case of the TNDM candidate gene *PLAGL1/ZAC1* [10]. Perhaps surprisingly, only a minority of imprinted genes are directly controlled by DNA methylation in this manner [40], and it is a common misconception that all imprinted genes are mono-allelically methylated. Most imprinted genes are controlled by indirect mechanisms which, however, are all ultimately reliant on an ICR which is determined by methylation. This is most obvious in the case of extensive imprinted gene clusters that come under the control of a single ICR. Knockout work in mice shows that deletion of a single such element results in the ablation of imprinting of multiple genes in cis in the cluster [41, 42]. A common mechanism for mono-allelic expression across a gene cluster appears to be via non-coding, antisense transcripts. Examples of this are the non-coding transcript *Air* in controlling imprinting of *Igf2r* [43], and the *Kcnq1ot1* transcript in controlling imprinting of the *Kcnq1* domain, including the Beckwith-Wiedemann syndrome gene *Cdkn1c* [41]. In these cases, some of the genes controlled are overlapped by the non-coding RNA, but

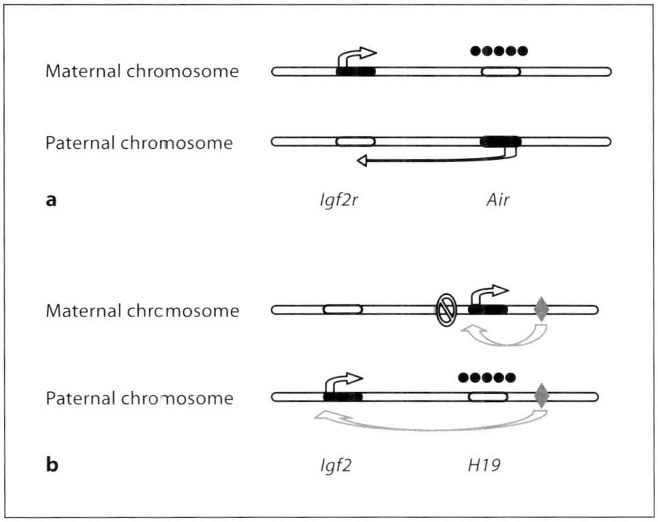

Fig. 1. Mechanisms of mono-allelic expression at imprinted genes. Two well-characterised mechanisms are illustrated. **a** Mono-allelic silencing by non-coding antisense RNA *(Air)* of the *Igf2r* gene. *Igf2r* is silenced on the paternal chromosome as a result of expression of the non-coding RNA *Air*, which transcribes through the *Igf2r* gene. Mono-allelic expression of *Air* is determined by the ICR which comprises dense DNA methylation (represented as filled circles) at the *Air* promoter; this methylation, which is restricted to the maternal chromosome, is established in female germ cells. **b** Mono-allelic silencing of *Igf2* by the action of an insulator element. The insulator upstream of the adjacent *H19* gene operates on the maternal chromosome to prevent downstream enhancers (grey diamonds) from interacting with the *Igf2* promoters. On the paternal allele, insulator function is eliminated by DNA methylation (deriving from sperm), resulting in silencing of *H19* and activation of *Igf2*.

others are not. It is not clear therefore what the mechanism of silencing is, other than it may ultimately involve repressive histone modifications, or what determines the boundary of the imprinted domain. A second, well-characterised mechanism involves allele-specific chromatin boundaries, as exemplified by the reciprocal imprinting of the closely linked *Igf2* and *H19* genes. A key component of this mechanism is the multifunctional protein CTCF, which creates a chromatin boundary between the *Igf2* and *H19* genes on the unmethylated maternal allele, thereby denying access of the *Igf2* gene promoters to enhancers downstream of *H19* [44, 45]. It is likely that additional levels of regulation overlay this elegant model, particularly for an imprinted gene of such pivotal importance as *Igf2* [46].

The reader might like to ponder that the notion of conflict between imprinted genes thus also extends to their regulation: the paternally expressed non-coding RNA *Air* accomplishes the silencing of the paternal allele of the *Igf2r* gene, and mechanisms governing maternal allele expression of *H19* ensure maternal allele silencing of *Igf2*.

Is imprinting all or nothing? Where there is direct DNA methylation-dependent silencing of a promoter, it is likely that imprinting of the associated gene is constitutive; there is little evidence that the dense regions of DNA methylation characteristic of ICRs can be significantly modulated during normal development to allow biallelic expression. If such a gene escapes imprinting in specific tissues, it is more likely that the gene possesses alternative promoters, where one or another promoter is not heavily methylated (as in the case of biallelic expression of *PLAGL1/ZAC1* in lymphocytes [47]). Hence, it is important to be aware of the detailed organisation of a gene and distribution of methylation. Conversely, where mechanisms of silencing are indirect there is likely to be more scope for the imprinting of a gene to vary during development, between tissues or during ageing, what might be termed 'leaky' imprinting or tissue-specific imprinted expression. Is tissue-specific imprinting of consequence? There are examples of exquisitely tissue-specific imprinting of real functional significance. Mono-allelic expression (paternal allele silencing) of *UBE3A,* the AS gene, is localised to highly specific neurons. Its ICR is about 500 kb away and imprinting is thought to be determined by a long-range antisense RNA [48]. Nevertheless, AS can develop from inactivating mutations in the maternal copy of *UBE3A*. For the gene *Gnas,* which encodes the stimulating G-protein subunit Gsα, relative silencing of the paternal allele is restricted to very few cell types, such as renal proximal tubules, adipocytes, the pituitary and thyroid glands [49, 50]. This highly restricted, tissue-specific imprinting is determined by a DNA methylation mark upstream of the authentic *Gnas* promoter; the *Gnas* promoter itself appears to be a conventional, constitutively unmethylated CpG island [51]. The fact that tissue-specific imprinting of *Gnas* is conserved between mouse and human suggests that it derives from a strong selective advantage; constitutive imprinting of *Gnas* may be too risky to have been favoured evolutionarily because of the involvement of Gsα in so many endocrine and homeostatic pathways. Tissue-specific imprinting of *GNAS* in humans accounts for the tissue-specific hormone resistance syndrome, pseudohypoparathyroidism type 1, caused by maternally inherited inactivating mutations in *GNAS*. In the case of the *Kcnq1* domain, many of the genes in the cluster display paternal allele silencing only in the placenta [52]. Interestingly, this placental-specific imprinting occurs in the mouse but not the orthologous human cluster [53], which might relate to differences in the relative importance of imprinting in the placenta in these species, perhaps as a function of litter size. It is conceivable that tissue-specific imprinted genes that rely on indirect and sometimes remote ICRs may be the most susceptible to environmental, nutritional or age-related modulations in imprinting.

Functions of Imprinted Genes in Metabolism

We have seen above that the control of fetal growth, via actions in the fetus or in the placenta, is a major arena for imprinted genes, and one which can be rationalised by a single explanation based on parental gene conflict. Imprinted genes do not cease to

Table 2. Imprinted genes with adult metabolic phenotypes in mice

Gene	Expressed allele	Null phenotype[1]	Ref.
Dlk1	paternal	increased adiposity, diet-induced obesity	70
Gnas[2]	maternal	obesity, insulin resistance, suppressed metabolic rate	57
Gnasxl[3]	paternal	leanness, insulin sensitivity, elevated metabolic rate	56
Grb10	maternal	reduced adiposity	76
Peg3	paternal	increased adiposity, suppressed metabolic rate, cold intolerant	77
Rasgrf1	paternal	impaired glucose tolerance, reduced β-cell mass	61

[1] Describes the effect of targeted disruption of the gene. Most effects relate to mice heterozygous for inactivating mutations, where the mutations are carried on the normally active allele. Homozygous mutants are expected to be similarly affected.
[2] *Gnas* is subject to tissue-restricted imprinting with silencing of paternal allele in a subset of tissues. This phenotype refers to heterozygotes with inactivating mutation on the maternal allele; therefore, those tissues with imprinted expression are deficient in *Gnas*. Paternal transmission of the mutation results in a distinct phenotype.
[3] *Gnasxl* encodes the Gsα variant XLαs.

be expressed at birth, however, and it is becoming increasingly evident that they have profound effects after birth that can persist into adulthood or even influence behaviours. The complex neuro-endocrine disorder Prader-Willi syndrome is a prime example that loss of imprinted genes can have severe and changing consequences for well-being in the infant and throughout life. Knockout studies in mice are also informative (table 2). Frequently observed amongst phenotypes are effects on adiposity, peripheral glucose sensitivity and metabolic rate. It is apparent that imprinted genes can operate across multiple physiological systems and influence the development or function of multiple endocrine axes; however, our knowledge of how imprinted genes act on adult metabolism is less well developed than our understanding of imprinting in fetal growth. This is compounded by the fact that many of these genes are also expressed during embryonic development and influence fetal growth, so it may be difficult to dissociate adult phenotypes from their consequences in utero, for example through IUGR, which might be responsible for programming adult metabolism. Furthermore, whereas there was an obvious asymmetry in the effects of paternally expressed and maternally expressed imprinted genes on fetal growth, metabolic phenotypes do not sort neatly in the same way.

Set against this uncertainty, a particularly illuminating example is provided by the *Gnas* locus. This complex imprinted domain encodes Gsα from the canonical *Gnas* transcript, whose expression is silenced on the paternal allele in a tissue-specific manner, including in adipose tissue. In addition, there is an overlapping transcript that codes for an elongated form of Gsα called 'extra large αs' (XLαs). Intriguingly, imprinting of the XLαs transcript is opposite to that of Gsα, such that it is only expressed from the paternal allele [54, 55]. Knockout studies have shown both Gsα and XLαs to be essential, but with strikingly different phenotypic consequences. Loss of maternally expressed Gsα leads to a complex perinatal phenotype, including enhanced birth weight, oedema and a high rate of lethality [49]; deficiency of XLαs is characterised by poor feeding, extreme leanness, acute hypoglycaemia, failure to thrive and markedly reduced survival [27]. This latter phenotype appears to meet well with expectations of the conflict hypothesis of a resource hungry, paternal gene. But it is in adults that the contrast in phenotypes becomes most remarkable. XLαs-null mice remain very lean throughout adult life as a result of enhanced metabolic rate, possibly owing to constitutively increased activity of the sympathetic nervous system towards adipose tissue [56]. The mutants have increased insulin sensitivity and glucose uptake, and a gene expression profile in adipose tissues consistent with increased sympathetic stimulation. In striking contrast, loss of maternal Gsα leads to obesity, impaired glucose tolerance and insulin resistance, and suppressed metabolic rate and sympathetic tone [57]. Thus it appears that notions of conflict and antagonism between oppositely imprinted genes can extend to adult physiology as well as to life in utero, and can exist within a single imprinted cluster.

Imprinting and the Pancreas

Several imprinted genes participate in the control of blood glucose homeostasis via actions in glucose-sensitive tissues and in the central nervous system. Fewer have yet been shown explicitly to affect the pancreas directly. TNDM provides a precedent that overexpression of a single imprinted locus can profoundly affect β-cell development or function, but in a transient manner. Given that TNDM is caused by LoI and overexpression of an imprinted gene, an attempt has been made in mice to model the disorder by expression of human *PLAGL1/ZAC1* (the TNDM candidate gene) using a large fragment transgene [58]. This resulted in a transgenic line that copiously expressed the human locus, and displayed hyperglycaemia in pups and a tendency to impaired glucose tolerance in adult mice. Notably, however, the neonatal transgenic mice are not deficient in insulin production in the same way as TNMD infants are. Studies of the transgenic embryos indicated a retarded development of the endocrine pancreas, with reduced expression of key endocrine determining transcription factors such as Pdx1, Ngn3 and Pax6 in the pancreas in mid gestation, associated with a reduction in cells expressing insulin and other endocrine hormones. Nevertheless, the precise molecular defects in TNDM (and in the mouse model) are still rather obscure and further studies are required: it is not clear how the TNDM β-cell is so compromised perinatally, but can recover within the first months of life, albeit within a lifelong potential for relapse to permanent diabetes. This might correspond to the presence of functionally distinct classes of β-cells in the fetal, neonatal and adult stages, consistent with waves of neogenesis and cell replacement [59].

Of the imprinted genes with an effect on the endocrine pancreas, currently the best studied is *Rasgrf1*. This paternally expressed imprinted gene encodes the Ras guanine nucleotide-releasing factor GRF1. Previous studies indicated GRF1 to be expressed predominantly in the brain, and knockout mice have delayed growth postnatally [60], probably as a result of reduced IGF1 levels. More recent analysis has identified a reduction in serum insulin, mildly impaired glucose tolerance, but isolated islets from *Rasgrf1*-null mice respond normally to glucose-stimulated insulin release [61]. There is a reduction in β-cell number as a result of reduced proliferation, at least around the weaning period (*Rasgrf1* is not expressed before birth). Islets respond poorly to stimulation by IGF1, with blunted activation of Akt and Erk phosphorylation, consistent with the established role of the IGF1 pathway as a regulator of β-cell mass. Interestingly, *Rasgrf1* is regulated by a distant ICR [62] which, as suggested above, could render this gene vulnerable to modulation through environmental effects or developmental programming events.

Imprinting and Diabetes Genes

There has been great recent interest in large-scale gene association studies to identify diabetes genes, for both type 1 and type 2 diseases [e.g., 63, 64]. Earlier work had suggested associations for type 2 diabetes mapping close to the TNDM interval, for example at 6q24-q27 in African-Americans [65], and a weak association of paternally derived alleles of 6q in Pima Indians [66]. However, a large case-control study specifically aimed at investigating an association of the TNDM interval with type 2 diabetes failed to find one [67]. Nonetheless, it will be of interest to assess whether known imprinted genes emerge from large gene association studies, whether parent-of-origin effects can be found, and whether imprinted genes do behave as sensitive targets for developmental programming of β-cell function and susceptibility to diabetes.

References

1 Reik W, Walter J: Genomic imprinting: parental influence on the genome. Nat Rev Genet 2001;2:21–32.

2 Solter D: Imprinting today: end of the beginning or beginning of the end? Cytogenet Genome Res 2006; 113:12–16.

3 Morison IM, Ramsay JP, Spencer HG: A census of mammalian imprinting. Trends Genet 2005;21: 457–465.

4 Constância M, Kelsey G, Reik W: Resourceful imprinting. Nature 2004;432:53–57.

5 Killian JK, Nolan CM, Wylie AA, Li T, Vu TH, Hoffman AR, Jirtle RL: Divergent evolution in M6P/IGF2R imprinting from the Jurassic to the Quaternary. Hum Mol Genet 2001;10:1721–1728.

6 Hatada I, Ohashi H, Fukushima Y, Kaneko Y, Inoue M, Komoto Y, Okada A, Ohishi S, Nabetani A, Morisaki H, Nakayama M, Niikawa N, Mukai T: An imprinted gene p57KIP2 is mutated in Beckwith-Wiedemann syndrome. Nat Genet 1996;14:171–173.

7 Kishino T, Lalande M, Wagstaff J: UBE3A/E6-AP mutations cause Angelman syndrome. Nat Genet 1997;15:70–73.
8 Matsuura T, Sutcliffe JS, Fang P, Galjaard RJ, Jiang YH, Benton CS, Rommens JM, Beaudet AL: De novo truncating mutations in E6-AP ubiquitin-protein ligase gene (UBE3A) in Angelman syndrome. Nat Genet 1997;15:74–77.
9 Temple IK, Shield JP: Transient neonatal diabetes, a disorder of imprinting. J Med Genet 2002;39:872–875.
10 Arima T, Drewell RA, Arney KL, Inoue J, Makita Y, Hata A, Oshimura M, Wake N, Surani MA: A conserved imprinting control region at the HYMAI/ZAC domain is implicated in transient neonatal diabetes mellitus. Hum Mol Genet 2001;10:1475–1483.
11 Mackay DJ, Coupe AM, Shield JP, Storr JN, Temple IK, Robinson DO: Relaxation of imprinted expression of ZAC and HYMAI in a patient with transient neonatal diabetes mellitus. Hum Genet 2002;110:139–144.
12 Tucker KL, Beard C, Dausmann J, Jackson-Grusby L, Laird PW, Lei H, Li E, Jaenisch R: Germ-line passage is required for establishment of methylation and expression patterns of imprinted but not of nonimprinted genes. Genes Dev 1996;10:1008–1020.
13 Gosden R, Trasler J, Lucifero D, Faddy M: Rare congenital disorders, imprinted genes, and assisted reproductive technology. Lancet 2003;361:1975–1977.
14 Gallou-Kabani C, Junien C: Nutritional epigenomics of metabolic syndrome: new perspective against the epidemic. Diabetes 2005;54:1899–1906.
15 Sinclair SK, Lea RG, Rees WD, Young LE: The developmental origins of health and disease: current theories and epigenetic mechanisms. Soc Reprod Fertil Suppl 2007;64:425–443.
16 Ogawa O, Eccles MR, Szeto J, McNoe LA, Yun K, Maw MA, Smith PJ, Reeve AE: Relaxation of insulin-like growth factor II gene imprinting implicated in Wilms' tumour. Nature 1993;362:749–751.
17 Rainier S, Johnson LA, Dobry CJ, Ping AJ, Grundy PE, Feinberg AP: Relaxation of imprinted genes in human cancer. Nature 1993;362:747–749.
18 Feinberg AP, Tycko B: The history of cancer epigenetics. Nat Rev Cancer 2004;4:143–153.
19 Abdollahi A, Pisarcik D, Roberts D, Weinstein J, Cairns P, Hamilton TC: LOT1 (PLAGL1/ZAC1), the candidate tumor suppressor gene at chromosome 6q24–25, is epigenetically regulated in cancer. J Biol Chem 2003;278:6041–6049.
20 Haig D, Graham C: Genomic imprinting and the strange case of the insulin-like growth factor II receptor. Cell 1991;64:1045–1046.
21 DeChiara TM, Robertson EJ, Efstratiadis A: Parental imprinting of the mouse insulin-like growth factor II gene. Cell 1991;64:849–859.
22 Leighton PA, Ingram RS, Eggenschwiler J, Efstratiadis A, Tilghman SM: Disruption of imprinting caused by deletion of the H19 gene region in mice. Nature 1995;375:34–39.
23 Wang ZQ, Fung MR, Barlow DP, Wagner EF: Regulation of embryonic growth and lysosomal targeting by the imprinted Igf2/Mpr gene. Nature 1994;372:464–467.
24 Wutz A, Theussl HC, Dausman J, Jaenisch R, Barlow DP, Wagner EF: Non-imprinted Igf2r expression decreases growth and rescues the Tme mutation in mice. Development 2001;128:1881–1887.
25 Thorvaldsen JL, Duran KL, Bartolomei MS: Deletion of the H19 differentially methylated domain results in loss of imprinted expression of H19 and Igf2. Genes Dev 1998;12:3693–3702.
26 Moore T, Haig D: Genomic imprinting in mammalian development: a parental tug-of-war. Trends Genet 1991;7:45–49.
27 Plagge A, Gordon E, Dean W, Boiani R, Cinti S, Peters J, Kelsey G: The imprinted signaling protein XL alpha s is required for postnatal adaptation to feeding. Nat Genet 2004;36:818–826.
28 Wilkins JF, Haig D: What good is genomic imprinting: the function of parent-specific gene expression. Nat Rev Genet 2003;4:359–368.
29 Haig D, Wharton R: Prader-Willi syndrome and the evolution of human childhood. Am J Hum Biol 2003;15:320–329.
30 Brown WM, Consedine NS: Just how happy is the happy puppet? An emotion signaling and kinship theory perspective on the behavioral phenotype of children with Angelman syndrome. Med Hypotheses 2004;63:377–385.
31 Hurst LD, McVean GT: Do we understand the evolution of genomic imprinting? Curr Opin Genet Dev 1998;8:701–708.
32 Schaefer CB, Ooi SK, Bestor TH, Bourc'his D: Epigenetic decisions in mammalian germ cells. Science 2007;316:398–399.
33 Kaneda M, Okano M, Hata K, Sado T, Tsujimoto N, Li E, Sasaki H: Essential role for de novo DNA methyltransferase Dnmt3a in paternal and maternal imprinting. Nature 2004;429:900–903.
34 Bourc'his D, Xu GL, Lin CS, Bollman B, Bestor TH: Dnmt3L and the establishment of maternal genomic imprints. Science 2001;294:2536–2539.
35 Hata K, Okano M, Lei H, Li E: Dnmt3L cooperates with the Dnmt3 family of de novo DNA methyltransferases to establish maternal imprints in mice. Development 2002;129:1983–1993.
36 Neumann B, Kubicka P, Barlow DP: Characteristics of imprinted genes. Nat Genet 1995;9:12–13.

37 Wood AJ, Roberts RG, Monk D, Moore GE, Schulz R, Oakey RJ: A screen for retrotransposed imprinted genes reveals an association between X chromosome homology and maternal germ-line methylation. PLoS Genet 2007;3:e20.

38 Reik W, Dean W, Walter J: Epigenetic reprogramming in mammalian development. Science 2001; 293:1089–1093.

39 Delaval K, Feil R: Epigenetic regulation of mammalian genomic imprinting. Curr Opin Genet Dev 2004;14:188–195.

40 Yatsuki H, Joh K, Higashimoto K, Soejima H, Arai Y, Wang Y, Hatada I, Obata Y, Morisaki H, Zhang Z, Nakagawachi T, Satoh Y, Mukai T: Domain regulation of imprinting cluster in Kip2/Lit1 subdomain on mouse chromosome 7F4/F5: large-scale DNA methylation analysis reveals that DMR-Lit1 is a putative imprinting control region. Genome Res 2002;12:1860–1870.

41 Fitzpatrick GV, Soloway PD, Higgins MJ: Regional loss of imprinting and growth deficiency in mice with a targeted deletion of KvDMR1. Nat Genet 2002;32:426–431.

42 Lin SP, Youngson N, Takada S, Seitz H, Reik W, Paulsen M, Cavaille J, Ferguson-Smith AC: Asymmetric regulation of imprinting on the maternal and paternal chromosomes at the Dlk1-Gtl2 imprinted cluster on mouse chromosome 12. Nat Genet 2003;35:97–102.

43 Sleutels F, Zwart R, Barlow DP: The non-coding Air RNA is required for silencing autosomal imprinted genes. Nature 2002;415:810–813.

44 Hark AT, Schoenherr CJ, Katz DJ, Ingram RS, Levorse JM, Tilghman SM: CTCF mediates methylation-sensitive enhancer-blocking activity at the H19/Igf2 locus. Nature 2000;405:486–489.

45 Bell AC, Felsenfeld G: Methylation of a CTCF-dependent boundary controls imprinted expression of the Igf2 gene. Nature 2000;405:482–485.

46 Murrell A, Heeson S, Reik W: Interaction between differentially methylated regions partitions the imprinted genes Igf2 and H19 into parent-specific chromatin loops. Nat Genet 2004;36:889–893.

47 Valleley EM, Cordery SF, Bonthron DT: Tissue-specific imprinting of the ZAC/PLAGL1 tumour suppressor gene results from variable utilization of monoallelic and biallelic promoters. Hum Mol Genet 2007;16:972–981.

48 Runte M, Hüttenhofer A, Gross S, Kiefmann M, Horsthemke B, Buiting K: The IC-SNURF-SNRPN transcript serves as a host for multiple small nucleolar RNA species and as an antisense RNA for UBE3A. Hum Mol Genet 2001;10:2687–2700.

49 Yu S, Yu D, Lee E, Eckhaus M, Lee R, Corria Z, Accili D, Westphal H, Weinstein LS: Variable and tissue-specific hormone resistance in heterotrimeric Gs protein alpha-subunit (Gsalpha) knockout mice is due to tissue-specific imprinting of the gsalpha gene. Proc Natl Acad Sci USA 1998;95:8715–8720.

50 Mantovani G, Ballare E, Giammona E, Beck-Peccoz P, Spada A: The gsalpha gene: predominant maternal origin of transcription in human thyroid gland and gonads. J Clin Endocrinol Metab 2002;87: 4736–4740.

51 Williamson CM, Ball ST, Nottingham WT, Skinner JA, Plagge A, Turner MD, Powles N, Hough T, Papworth D, Fraser WD, Maconochie M, Peters J: A cis-acting control region is required exclusively for the tissue-specific imprinting of Gnas. Nat Genet 2004; 36:894–899.

52 Lewis A, Mitsuya K, Umlauf D, Smith P, Dean W, Walter J, Higgins M, Feil R, Reik W: Imprinting on distal chromosome 7 in the placenta involves repressive histone methylation independent of DNA methylation. Nat Genet 2004;36:1291–1295.

53 Monk D, Arnaud P, Apostolidou S, Hills FA, Kelsey G, Stanier P, Feil R, Moore GE: Limited evolutionary conservation of imprinting in the human placenta. Proc Natl Acad Sci USA 2006;103:6623–6628.

54 Hayward BE, Kamiya M, Strain L, Moran V, Campbell R, Hayashizaki Y, Bonthron DT: The human GNAS1 gene is imprinted and encodes distinct paternally and biallelically expressed G proteins. Proc Natl Acad Sci USA 1998;95:10038–10043.

55 Peters J, Wroe SF, Wells CA, Miller HJ, Bodle D, Beechey CV, Williamson CM, Kelsey G: A cluster of oppositely imprinted transcripts at the Gnas locus in the distal imprinting region of mouse chromosome 2. Proc Natl Acad Sci USA 1999;96:3830–3835.

56 Xie T, Plagge A, Gavrilova O, Pack S, Jou W, Lai EW, Frontera M, Kelsey G, Weinstein LS: The alternative stimulatory G protein alpha-subunit XLalphas is a critical regulator of energy and glucose metabolism and sympathetic nerve activity in adult mice. J Biol Chem 2006;281:18989–18999.

57 Yu S, Gavrilova O, Chen H, Lee R, Liu J, Pacak K, Parlow AF, Quon MJ, Reitman ML, Weinstein LS: Paternal versus maternal transmission of a stimulatory G-protein alpha subunit knockout produces opposite effects on energy metabolism. J Clin Invest 2000;105:615–623.

58 Ma D, Shield JP, Dean W, Leclerc I, Knauf C, Burcelin R R, Rutter GA, Kelsey G: Impaired glucose homeostasis in transgenic mice expressing the human transient neonatal diabetes mellitus locus, TNDM. J Clin Invest 2004;114:339–348.

59 Scaglia L, Cahill CJ, Finegood DT, Bonner-Weir S: Apoptosis participates in the remodeling of the endocrine pancreas in the neonatal rat. Endocrinology 1997;138:1736–1741.

60 Itier JM, Tremp GL, Léonard JF, Multon MC, Ret G, Schweighoffer F, Tocqué B, Bluet-Pajot MT, Cormier V, Dautry F: Imprinted gene in postnatal growth role. Nature 1998;393:125–126.

61 Font de Mora J, Esteban LM, Burks DJ, Núñez A, Garcés C, García-Barrado MJ, Iglesias-Osma MC, Moratinos J, Ward JM, Santos E: Ras-GRF1 signaling is required for normal beta-cell development and glucose homeostasis. EMBO J 2003;22:3039–3049.

62 Plass C, Shibata H, Kalcheva I, Mullins L, Kotelevtseva N, Mullins J, Kato R, Sasaki H, Hirotsune S, Okazaki Y, Held WA, Hayashizaki Y, Chapman VM: Identification of Grf1 on mouse chromosome 9 as an imprinted gene by RLGS-M. Nat Genet 1996;14:106–109.

63 Hakonarson H, Grant SF, Bradfield JP, Marchand L, Kim CE, Glessner JT, Grabs R, Casalunovo T, Taback SP, Frackelton EC, Lawson ML, Robinson LJ, Skraban R, Lu Y, Chiavacci RM, Stanley CA, Kirsch SE, Rappaport EF, Orange JS, Monos DS, Devoto M, Qu HQ, Polychronakos C: A genome-wide association study identifies KIAA0350 as a type 1 diabetes gene. Nature 2007;448:591–594.

64 Sladek R, Rocheleau G, Rung J, Dina C, Shen L, Serre D, Boutin P, Vincent D, Belisle A, Hadjadj S, Balkau B, Heude B, Charpentier G, Hudson TJ, Montpetit A, Pshezhetsky AV, Prentki M, Posner BI, Balding DJ, Meyre D, Polychronakos C, Froguel P: A genome-wide association study identifies novel risk loci for type 2 diabetes. Nature 2007;445: 881–885.

65 Sale MM, Freedman BI, Langefeld CD, Williams AH, Hicks PJ, Colicigno CJ, Beck SR, Brown WM, Rich SS, Bowden DW: A genome-wide scan for type 2 diabetes in African-American families reveals evidence for a locus on chromosome 6q. Diabetes 2004;53:830–837.

66 Lindsay RS, Kobes S, Knowler WC, Bennett PH, Hanson RL: Genome-wide linkage analysis assessing parent-of-origin effects in the inheritance of type 2 diabetes and BMI in Pima Indians. Diabetes 2001;50:2850–2857.

67 Gloyn AL, Mackay DJ, Weedon MN, McCarthy MI, Walker M, Hitman G, Knight BA, Owen KR, Hattersley AT, Frayling TM: Assessment of the role of common genetic variation in the transient neonatal diabetes mellitus (TNDM) region in type 2 diabetes: a comparative genomic and tagging single nucleotide polymorphism approach. Diabetes 2006; 55:2272–2276.

68 Guillemot F, Caspary T, Tilghman SM, Copeland NG, Gilbert DJ, Jenkins NA, Anderson DJ, Joyner AL, Rossant J, Nagy A: Genomic imprinting of Mash2, a mouse gene required for trophoblast development. Nat Genet 1995;9:235–242.

69 Takahashi K, Kobayashi T, Kanayama N: p57(Kip2) regulates the proper development of labyrinthine and spongiotrophoblasts. Mol Hum Reprod 2000;6: 1019–1025.

70 Moon YS, Smas CM, Lee K, Villena JA, Kim KH, Yun EJ, Sul HS: Mice lacking paternally expressed Pref-1/Dlk1 display growth retardation and accelerated adiposity. Mol Cell Biol 2002;22:5585–5592.

71 Charalambous M, Smith FM, Bennett WR, Crew TE, Mackenzie F, Ward A: Disruption of the imprinted Grb10 gene leads to disproportionate overgrowth by an Igf2-independent mechanism. Proc Natl Acad Sci USA 2003;100:8292–8297.

72 Lefebvre L, Viville S, Barton SC, Ishino F, Keverne EB, Surani MA: Abnormal maternal behaviour and growth retardation associated with loss of the imprinted gene Mest. Nat Genet 1998;20:163–169.

73 Curley JP, Barton S, Surani A, Keverne EB: Coadaptation in mother and infant regulated by a paternally expressed imprinted gene. Proc Biol Sci 2004; 271:1303–1309.

74 Salas M, John R, Saxena A, Barton S, Frank D, Fitzpatrick G, Higgins MJ, Tycko B: Placental growth retardation due to loss of imprinting of Phlda2. Mech Dev 2004;121:1199–1210.

75 Varrault A, Gueydan C, Delalbre A, Bellmann A, Houssami S, Aknin C, Severac D, Chotard L, Kahli M, Le Digarcher A, Pavlidis P, Journot L: Zac1 regulates an imprinted gene network critically involved in the control of embryonic growth. Dev Cell 2006; 11:711–722.

76 Smith FM, Holt LJ, Garfield AS, Charalambous M, Koumanov F, Perry M, Bazzani R, Sheardown SA, Hegarty BD, Lyons RJ, Cooney GJ, Daly RJ, Ward A: Mice with a disruption of the imprinted Grb10 gene exhibit altered body composition, glucose homeostasis and insulin signalling during post-natal life. Mol Cell Biol 2007;27:5871–5886.

77 Curley JP, Pinnock SB, Dickson SL, Thresher R, Miyoshi N, Surani MA, Keverne EB: Increased body fat in mice with a targeted mutation of the paternally expressed imprinted gene Peg3. FASEB J 2005; 19:1302–1304.

Dr. Gavin Kelsey
Laboratory of Developmental Genetics and Imprinting
The Babraham Institute
Cambridge CB22 3AT (UK)
Tel. +44 1223 496332, Fax +44 1223 496022, E-Mail gavin.kelsey@bbsrc.ac.uk

Shield JPH, Scharfmann R (eds): Development of the Pancreas and Neonatal Diabetes.
Endocr Dev. Basel, Karger, 2007, vol 12, pp 113–123

Imprinting in Human Disease with Special Reference to Transient Neonatal Diabetes and Beckwith-Wiedemann Syndrome

I. Karen Temple

Wessex Clinical Genetics Academic Group, Division of Human Genetics,
University of Southampton, Southampton, UK

Abstract

There are at least 6 well-studied imprinting domains on human autosomes. Each domain is under the regulatory control of an 'imprinting centre' that harbours a differentially methylated region. A number of molecular mechanisms result in differential silencing of some genes within these domains and gene expression is tightly regulated in normal individuals. However, this makes them vulnerable to naturally occurring genetic and epigenetic aberrations. Nine recognisable developmental syndromes have been described due to abnormalities within these 5 domains: transient neonatal diabetes (TND; at 6q24); Beckwith-Wiedemann syndrome (BWS) and Silver-Russell syndrome (at 11p15.5; 2 imprinted domains); maternal and paternal uniparental disomy syndromes (at 14q32); Angelman and Prader-Willi syndromes (at 15q11–13), and pseudohypoparathyroidism type 1b (at 20q12–13). Furthermore, it is now recognised that involvement at multiple domains can occur simultaneously and result in what has been described as the hypomethylation syndrome. TND and BWS are discussed in more detail as examples of imprinting disorders.

The Clinical Phenotypes

Transient neonatal diabetes (TND) related to 6q24 is a condition which presents classically within the first week of life with growth retardation and hyperglycaemia. Insulin therapy is required for normalisation of blood glucose in most patients and weight gain and apparent remission occur by 3 months (range 1–18 months) [1, 2]. Subsequent growth is normal. A significant proportion of affected individuals develop diabetes in later life with a mean age of 14 years [1]. While most of the literature on this type of TND stresses the diabetic aspects of the disorder, there are non-diabetic manifestations in some patients including umbilical hernia, macroglossia and learning difficulties.

In contrast, the Beckwith-Wiedemann syndrome (BWS) [3] is defined in terms of the somatic features which similarly present at birth and characteristically include the triad of overgrowth, umbilical abnormalities and macroglossia. Hemihypertrophy, ear creases and an increased risk of Wilms' tumour are significant features. Abnormal glycaemic control in the form of early-onset transient hypoglycaemia is a variable, although recognised feature of the condition.

There are therefore intriguing parallels and opposites in the clinical presentation of both conditions. Furthermore, both are due to altered expression of imprinted genes, which was uncovered by demonstrating uniparental disomy (UPD), the inheritance of a chromosome pair from only one parent with no contribution from the other. In TND, paternal UPD of chromosome 6 was identified in the first 2 cases [4]. In BWS, paternal partial UPD of chromosome 11 was identified [5]. This led to the hypothesis that the symptoms were due to aberrant expression of imprinted genes on the respective chromosomes, which has subsequently been shown to be the case.

Epigenetic Regulation of Imprinted Genes

Imprinted genes differ from most gene pairs in that only one gene of the pair is expressed and the other is silenced in a pattern that reflects the parent from which they originated. This comes about because expression patterns of most of the imprinted genes identified so far are under the control of regulatory regions of DNA called 'imprinting centres' which contain, in part, DNA which has been chemically 'marked'. The best-characterised biochemical mechanism is DNA methylation where DNA is chemically modified by methylation of cytosine nucleotides. For any one imprinted locus the 'marking' consistently occurs in either the developing sperm or ova such that the regions of DNA are able to resist the normal resetting of gene regulation that occurs soon after fertilisation. It results in a primary region of differential methylation in the developing fetus (called a DMR) on either the copy derived from the oocyte (the maternal allele) or the copy derived from the sperm (the paternal allele). It is of interest that there are more imprinted loci with oocyte-derived methylation 'marks', i.e. DMRs where the methylation is present on the maternal allele and not the paternal allele, than with sperm-derived 'marks', i.e. where differential methylation is on the paternal allele and not the maternal allele.

The control centres work in conjunction with a variety of different molecules and processes to achieve differential gene expression of some of the surrounding genes. The term 'epigenetics' is used to describe this phenomenon whereby gene expression is reversibly silenced/activated independent of change to gene structure.

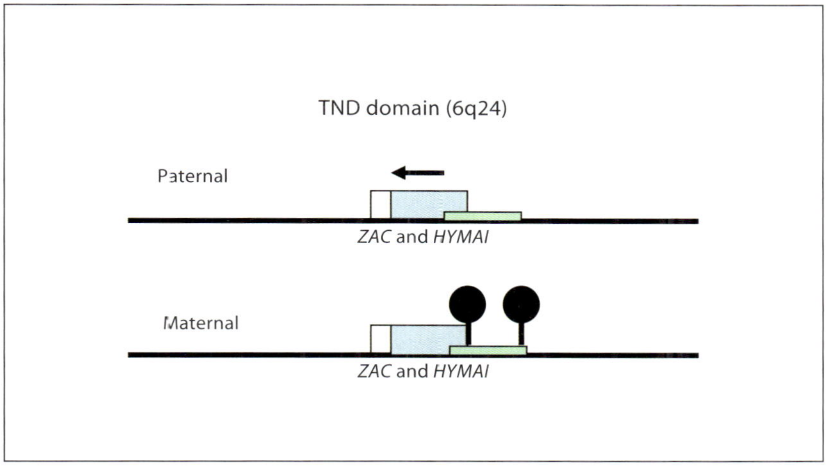

Fig. 1. Showing the TND domain at 6q24 with paternal expression of *ZAC* and *HYMAI*. The TND DMR is located in the promoter of both genes and the maternally methylated allele is associated with gene silencing in cis.

One of the simplest models is where the DMR lies within the promoter of a gene and the methylated copy is silenced (fig. 1). This is the case at the TND locus.

The Transient Neonatal Diabetes Imprinted Domain

At 6q24 there are two known imprinted genes, *ZAC* and *HYMAI* (fig. 1). *ZAC* codes for a zinc finger protein that localises to the nucleus and is a transcription factor. It is an inhibitor of cell proliferation inducing both apoptosis and cell cycle arrest [6]. *HYMAI* codes for an RNA gene of unknown function [7]. The exact relationship between *ZAC* and *HYMAI* is not understood, but both genes are expressed on the paternal allele and silenced on the maternal allele and have a common promoter region. The TND DMR overlaps exon 1 of both genes. Varrault et al. [8] showed that the DMR had promoter activity when it was unmethylated. The DMR is methylated on the maternal allele and unmethylated on the paternal allele. Arima et al. [9] have recently provided convincing evidence showing that this region is the likely imprinting centre for the domain. They showed that it confers differential expression of *ZAC* and *HYMAI* in mice [9]. In conclusion, differential methylation at the TND DMR results in paternal expression of *ZAC* and *HYMAI*.

The 11p15.5 locus implicated in BWS is more complex and contains two domains 280 kb apart.

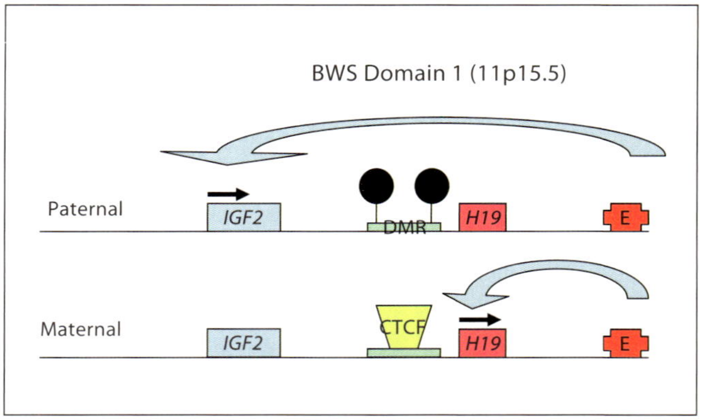

Fig. 2. Showing domain 1 of the BWS locus at 11p15.5. There is paternal expression of *IGF2* and maternal expression of *H19*. The DMR is paternally methylated. CCCTC insulator protein can only bind the non-methylated DMR and it insulates *IGF2* from its downstream enhancer.

The Beckwith-Wiedemann Imprinted Domain 1: *H19/IGF2*

Domain 1 has 2 reciprocally imprinted genes: *IGF2,* which is a potent fetal growth factor and is highly expressed in mesodermal and endodermal tissues, and *H19,* which is a non-coding RNA gene (fig. 2). *IGF2* and *H19* compete for the same enhancer and expression of both genes depends on a DMR that is paternally methylated. The CCCTC-binding factor (CTCF), an insulator molecule, binds the unmethylated maternal DMR, which creates a chromatin boundary preventing *IGF2* from binding to its downstream enhancer. Thus, *IGF2* is not expressed from the maternal allele, while *H19* is. On the paternal allele, methylation of the DMR means that CTCF does not bind it and so enhancers can bind *IGF2* promoters, which results in the expression of *IGF2* from the paternal allele. *H19* is not expressed on the paternal copy, probably due to an extension of methylation to include part of its promoter.

In conclusion, differential methylation at the *IGF2/H19* DMR results in reciprocal expression of *IGF2* from the paternally inherited allele and expression of *H19* from the maternally inherited allele.

The Beckwith-Wiedemann Imprinted Domain 2: KvDMR

Centromeric to the *H19/IGF2* DMR is a second imprinted domain regulated by an imprinting centre which harbours a DMR called KvDMR (fig. 3). This is methylated on the maternal allele and the exact way in which genes in the domain are differentially silenced is not certain [10]. KvDMR is within the promoter of a non-coding an-

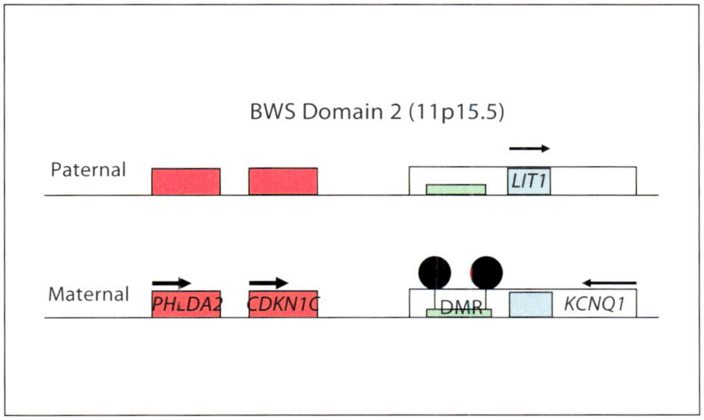

Fig. 3. Showing domain 2 of the BWS locus at 11p15.5. The DMR is maternally methylated. *LIT1* is expressed from the paternal allele only and is associated with silencing of *CDKN1C* and *PHLDA2* on the paternal allele. Methylation of the DMR is associated with expression of *CDKN1C* and *PHLDA2.*

tisense RNA gene called *LIT1 (KCNQ1OT1)* which itself is within an intron of a multi-exon gene called *KCNQ1.* This latter gene codes for a potassium channel that is not thought to contribute to the BWS phenotype. It is imprinted in some but not all tissues and in those tissues it is expressed from the maternal allele. *LIT1* is paternally expressed and maternally repressed by the differential methylation and may be involved in paternal silencing of genes in cis within the domain. However, it is not clear if it has a direct effect on transcription of nearby genes or whether the regulatory region harbours sites for insulators/enhancers as at *H19.* One of the protein-coding genes within the domain is *CDKN1C,* which is a growth restrictor and has a negative regulatory role on cell proliferation. Another gene in the domain is *PHLDA2,* which is important in placental growth. Both these genes are silenced on the allele inherited from the father (paternal allele). On the maternal methylated allele, *LIT1* expression is repressed and *CDKN1C* and *PHLDA2* are expressed.

In conclusion, therefore, differential methylation at the KvDMR results in maternal expression of *CDKN1C* and paternal expression of *LIT1.*

Characteristics of Imprinted Genes

The results of these molecular processes are domains within which are genes that have differentially expressed copies and where the pattern is dependent on the parent they have most recently been exposed to, i.e. imprinted genes. The controlling centres impact on more than one neighbouring gene and can act either to silence or activate an allele. As a result, imprinted genes tend to occur in clusters or domains where the boundaries are set by the physical distance of influence of the controlling centre.

They can act over distances of more than a megabase. Control of these genes is exquisitely regulated and may be different in different tissues.

Imprinted genes comprise only a small proportion of human genes [approximately 80 have been identified (http://www.geneimprint.com) with approximately half showing maternal and half paternal expression] [11]. Imprinted genes identified so far do not have a common function, although some of the most well-studied protein-coding genes are involved in growth, either as cell cycle inhibitors *(CDKN1C)* and tumour suppressors *(ZAC)*, or as growth factors *(IGF2* and *DLK1)*.

Imprinting Disorders in Humans

There are at least 6 known imprinting domains in human autosomes where aberrant expression of genes is responsible for recognisable developmental syndromes. The following 9 syndromes have been described due to abnormalities within these 6 domains: TND (at 6q24); BWS and Silver-Russell syndrome (at 11p15.5; 2 imprinted loci); maternal and paternal UPD syndromes (at 14q32); Angelman and Prader-Willi syndromes (at 15q11–13); pseudohypoparathyroidism type 1b (at 20q12–13), and multiple loci involved in the hypomethylation syndrome. This list does not include chromosome 7 where there are at least 3 known imprinted domains in humans (*GRB10* at 7p21; *Peg10/SGCE* at 7q21; *PEG1/MEST* at 7q32); however, it is not known which, if any, is responsible for the short stature phenotype seen in maternal UPD of chromosome 7.

Mechanisms of Disease in Human Imprinting Disorders – Chromosome Rearrangements and Epigenetic Mutations

It is not surprising that mono-allelic expression makes imprinted genes vulnerable to genetic rearrangements and epigenetic mutation. There are therefore many classical chromosome rearrangements, such as duplications and deletions that can result in abnormal expression of imprinted genes, the main difference being that there is usually a parent-of-origin effect. However, for imprinting disorders aberrant epigenetic control is an alternative mechanism resulting in abnormal gene expression (table 1).

6q24-Related Transient Neonatal Diabetes

There are 3 mechanisms that have accounted for all cases with 6q24-related TND to date [1, 2]: (1) paternal UPD of chromosome 6 (40%), (2) a paternally inherited duplication involving the TND locus at 6q24 (40%) and (3) loss of methylation (LOM), on

Table 1. Genetic and epigenetic causes of 6q24-related TND and BWS

Mechanism of disease	Transient neonatal diabetes related to 6q24	Beckwith-Wiedemann syndrome
Chromosome duplication	paternal; 6q24; 40%	paternal; 11p15.5; 1% [18]
Chromosome deletion	–	maternal microdeletion of *H19* DMR [16] and maternal microdeletion of *LIT1* [10]
Uniparental disomy	paternal chromosome 6; 40% (usually isodisomy and involving the whole chromosome)	partial paternal isodisomy of chromosome 11 involving 11p15.5; 20% [18]
Loss of methylation	LOM at TND DMR; 20%	LOM at KvDMR; 50% [18]
Gain of methylation	–	gain of methylation at *H19* DMR; maternal allele; 2–7% [13]
Genetic mutation	–	mutations in *CDKN1C;* 10% [18]
Other	3% with no explanation	10–20% no cause detected

the maternally derived allele, at the TND DMR (20%). Each mechanism results in overexpression of *ZAC* and *HYMAI,* either because there are two paternal copies or because the imprinting control has been lost by loss of the epigenetic signal (LOM). It is not clear exactly how overexpression of *ZAC* results in the phenotype. Work by Ma et al. [12] in the TND mouse has shown that overexpression of *ZAC* is associated with reduced pancreatic β-cell mass at birth. This would be compatible with the low insulin levels measured in affected neonates. Ma et al. [12] showed that in mice there follows a period of β-cell proliferation after birth which may explain the transient nature of the disorder. However, further work is required to understand the pathogenesis and why diabetes recurs later in life.

Beckwith-Wiedemann Syndrome

Patients with BWS have been reported with chromosome rearrangements or epigenetic aberrations involving either domain 1, domain 2 or both [13]. The relationship between the 2 domains is not fully understood but it seems unlikely to be coincidental that 2 complimentary and opposing domains are adjacent and abnormality of both can result in the same condition. There is evidence that epigenetic aberrations at domain 2 impacts on expression of genes in domain 1 but the exact mechanism is not yet explained [13].

Domain 1

Genetic aberrations that result in overexpression of *IGF2* are associated with BWS [14]. Rare cases (approximately 1%) of paternal duplications of 11p15.5 and maternal microdeletions involving *H19* DMR are reported [15]. Paternal UPD of chromosome 11 is more common and seen in about 20% of sporadic patients with BWS. In UPD cases, it is usually segmental and often mosaic. Complete paternal UPD of chromosome 11 does occur but is rare and often results in fetal death [16].

Epigenetic mutations are described and include maternal gain of methylation at the *H19* DMR in approximately 5% of cases. BWS patients with domain 1 abnormalities are at increased risk of Wilms' tumour but have a lower incidence of umbilical abnormalities than patients with domain 2 defects [13].

Domain 2

In domain 2, reduced/absent expression of *CDKN1C* leads to a BWS phenotype. The commonest cause accounting for 50% of cases with BWS is maternal LOM at the KvDMR that results in reduced expression of *CDKN1C* [14]. Likewise, maternally inherited chromosome translocations or deletions that delete KvDMR have a similar effect [10]. Approximately 10% of BWS cases have a DNA mutation within *CDKN1C.* However, these account for almost 40% of familial cases and result in an autosomal dominant pattern of inheritance but with symptoms of BWS only when the mutation is inherited from a mother [17].

In summary, genetic and epigenetic aberrations that result in overexpression of *IGF2* or reduced expression of *CDKN1C* cause the BWS phenotype.

It has recently been recognised [18] that the Silver-Russell syndrome, a condition characterised by pre- and postnatal growth retardation with relative sparing of the head and associated features such as triangular facial shape, hemihypertrophy, 5th finger clinodactyly, early puberty, hypoglycaemia and genital abnormalities, is caused by reduced expression of *IGF2.* The mechanisms underlying the condition so far described include chromosomal rearrangements such as maternal duplication of 11p15.5 [19], and epigenetic aberrations, most commonly LOM at the *H19* DMR [18].

Overlap Syndromes – The Hypomethylation Syndrome

The differences and similarities between BWS and TND have been noted for several years. It was Arima et al. [20] who first demonstrated that the promoter of *LIT1* contained binding sites for *ZAC* and provided evidence that *ZAC* may influence *CDKN1C* expression. Subsequently, Varrault et al. [21] have shown that *ZAC* is an important member of an imprinting gene network and has a direct impact on expression of several imprinted genes. It is possible, therefore, that imprinted genes are part of a common cellular pathway responsible for the overlap in clinical features.

However, it has recently become apparent that the underlying cause of epigenetic aberrations such as LOM may influence more than one loci simultaneously. Mackay et al. [22] showed that 2 patients, presenting with TND due to LOM at 6q24, also had mosaic LOM at KvDMR. Both are maternally methylated loci and they proposed a common underlying cause affecting at least two independent loci. One of the patients had a much larger umbilical hernia than is usually seen in TND cases suggesting there were overlapping clinical features. Subsequently, Mackay et al. [23] showed that LOM was more generalised and could affect several maternally methylated imprinted loci. Seven of 12 patients presenting with TND due to LOM at 6q24 had mosaic LOM at variable imprinted loci. The phenotypes were more variable in these patients and, although numbers were small, there was evidence that such patients had a higher incidence of other congenital abnormalities and a higher birth weight than was seen in TND cases due to other mechanisms. In the same month, Rossignol et al. [24] reported that a proportion of BWS patients with LOM at KvDMR had LOM at other loci. Some of these patients had been conceived using artificial reproductive techniques and the authors hypothesised that LOM at multiple locations may be a result of environmental influences. Further investigation is warranted and it is possible that new imprinting syndromes will emerge dependent on the extent and number of loci involved.

Genetic Counselling for Transient Neonatal Diabetes and Beckwith-Wiedemann Syndrome

It follows that prior to offering genetic counselling it is important that the underlying molecular mechanism is identified, as risks vary considerably. Chromosome rearrangements can be de novo or inherited and parental chromosomes must always be investigated. In imprinting disorders, risks for offspring will depend on which parent is the carrier. For example, the offspring of a father with a duplication of 6q24 will have a 50% risk of inheriting TND, while the offspring of a mother with a similar duplication will not be at risk of developing TND despite having a 50% chance of inheriting the duplication. Similarly, genetic mutations of *CDKN1C* cause BWS only if inherited from the mother and therefore can seem to skip generations.

Risks for sibs and offspring of individuals with epigenetic aberrations resulting in loss or gain of methylation are hard to predict at the present time but caution is required. While it has been assumed that most are sporadic, this is not always the case and recurrence has been reported in sibs with TND due to LOM in the absence of a demonstrable microdeletion [pers. commun.]. It should be recognised that some techniques used to identify abnormal methylation ratios between alleles may fail to distinguish between a microdeletion and an epigenetic modification and this should be considered. Furthermore, the discovery of a generalised hypomethylation syndrome with multiple affected imprinted loci means that an affected sib may have a different and more severe phenotype depending on which loci are involved and to what extent tissues are involved.

Conclusion

Imprinted genes are a small subset of genes that are differentially expressed dependent on the parent of origin. Complex molecular silencing mechanisms are associated with differential epigenetic modification and this makes them particularly vulnerable to genetic rearrangements and epigenetic aberrations. TND and BWS are examples of human disorders due to deranged expression of genes within the imprinting domains at 6q24 and 11p15.5.

References

1 Temple IK, Gardner RJ, Mackay DJ, Barber JC, Robinson DO, Shield JP: Transient neonatal diabetes: widening the understanding of the etiopathogenesis of diabetes. Diabetes 2000;49:1359–1366.

2 Cave H, Polak M, Drunat S, Denamur E, Czernichow P: Refinement of the 6q chromosomal region implicated in transient neonatal diabetes. Diabetes 2000;49:108–113.

3 Elliott M, Bayly R, Cole T, Temple IK, Maher ER: Clinical features and natural history of Beckwith-Wiedemann syndrome: presentation of 74 new cases. Clin Genet 1994;46:168–174.

4 Temple IK, James RS, Crolla JA, Sitch FL, Jacobs PA, Howell WM, Betts P, Baum JD, Shield JP: An imprinted gene(s) for diabetes? Nat Genet 1995;9:110–112.

5 Henry I, Bonaiti-Pellie C, Chehensse V, Beldjord C, Schwartz C, Utermann G, Junien C: Uniparental paternal disomy in a genetic cancer-predisposing syndrome. Nature 1991;351:665–667.

6 Varrault A, Ciani E, Apiou F, Bilanges B, Hoffmann A, Pantaloni C, Bockaert J, Spengler D, Journot L: hZAC encodes a zinc finger protein with antiproliferative properties and maps to a chromosomal region frequently lost in cancer. Proc Natl Acad Sci USA 1998;95:8835–8840.

7 Arima T, Drewell RA, Oshimura M, Wake N, Surani MA: A novel imprinted gene, HYMAI, is located within an imprinted domain on human chromosome 6 containing ZAC. Genomics 2000;67:248–255.

8 Varrault A, Bilanges B, Mackay DJ, Basyuk E, Ahr B, Fernandez C, Robinson DO, Bockaert J, Journot L: Characterization of the methylation-sensitive promoter of the imprinted ZAC gene supports its role in transient neonatal diabetes mellitus. J Biol Chem 2001;276:18653–18656.

9 Arima T, Yamasaki K, John RM, Kato K, Sakumi K, Nakabeppu Y, Wake N, Kono T: The human HYMAI/PLAGL1 differentially methylated region acts as an imprint control region in mice. Genomics 2006;88:650–658.

10 Niemitz EL, DeBaun MR, Fallon J, Murakami K, Kugoh H, Oshimura M, Feinberg AP: Microdeletion of LIT1 in familial Beckwith-Wiedemann syndrome. Am J Hum Genet 2004;75:844–849.

11 Wood AJ, Oakey RJ: Genomic imprinting in mammals: emerging themes and established theories. PLoS Genet 2006;2:e147.

12 Ma D, Shield JP, Dean W, Leclerc I, Knauf C, Burcelin RR, Rutter GA, Kelsey G: Impaired glucose homeostasis in transgenic mice expressing the human transient neonatal diabetes mellitus locus, TNDM. J Clin Invest 2004;114:339–348.

13 Engel JR, Smallwood A, Harper A, Higgins MJ, Oshimura M, Reik W, Schofield PN, Maher ER: Epigenotype-phenotype correlations in Beckwith-Wiedemann syndrome. J Med Genet 2000;37:921–926.

14 Diaz-Meyer N, Day CD, Khatod K, Maher ER, Cooper W, Reik W, Junien C, Graham G, Algar E, Der Kaloustian VM, Higgins MJ: Silencing of CDKN1C (p57KIP2) is associated with hypomethylation at KvDMR1 in Beckwith-Wiedemann syndrome. J Med Genet 2003;40:797–801.

15 Sparago A, Cerrato F, Vernucci M, Ferrero GB, Silengo MC, Riccio A: Microdeletions in the human H19 DMR result in loss of IGF2 imprinting and Beckwith-Wiedemann syndrome. Nat Genet 2004; 36:958–960.
16 Cooper WN, Curley R, Macdonald F, Maher ER: Mitotic recombination and uniparental disomy in Beckwith-Wiedemann syndrome. Genomics 2007; 89:613–617.
17 Weksberg R, Shuman C, Smith AC: Beckwith-Wiedemann syndrome. Am J Med Genet C Semin Med Genet 2005;137:12–23.
18 Gicquel C, Rossignol S, Cabrol S, Houang M, Steunou V, Barbu V, Danton F, Thibaud N, Le MM, Burglen L, Bertrand AM, Netchine I, Le BY: Epimutation of the telomeric imprinting center region on chromosome 11p15 in Silver-Russell syndrome. Nat Genet 2005;37:1003–1007.
19 Eggermann T, Meyer E, Obermann C, Heil I, Schuler H, Ranke MB, Eggermann K, Wollmann HA: Is maternal duplication of 11p15 associated with Silver-Russell syndrome? J Med Genet 2005;42:e26.
20 Arima T, Kamikihara T, Hayashida T, Kato K, Inoue T, Shirayoshi Y, Oshimura M, Soejima H, Mukai T, Wake N: ZAC, LIT1 (KCNQ1OT1) and p57KIP2 (CDKN1C) are in an imprinted gene network that may play a role in Beckwith-Wiedemann syndrome. Nucleic Acids Res 2005;33:2650–2660.
21 Varrault A, Gueydan C, Delalbre A, Bellmann A, Houssami S, Aknin C, Severac D, Chotard L, Kahli M, Le DA, Pavlidis P, Journot L: Zac1 regulates an imprinted gene network critically involved in the control of embryonic growth. Dev Cell 2006;11: 711–722.
22 Mackay DJ, Hahnemann JM, Boonen SE, Poerksen S, Bunyan DJ, White HE, Durston VJ, Thomas NS, Robinson DO, Shield JP, Clayton-Smith J, Temple IK: Epimutation of the TNDM locus and the Beckwith-Wiedemann syndrome centromeric locus in individuals with transient neonatal diabetes mellitus. Hum Genet 2006;119:179–184.
23 Mackay DJ, Boonen SE, Clayton-Smith J, Goodship J, Hahnemann JM, Kant SG, Njolstad PR, Robin NH, Robinson DO, Siebert R, Shield JP, White HE, Temple IK: A maternal hypomethylation syndrome presenting as transient neonatal diabetes mellitus. Hum Genet 2006;120:262–269.
24 Rossignol S, Steunou V, Chalas C, Kerjean A, Rigolet M, Viegas-Pequignot E, Jouannet P, Le BY, Gicquel C: The epigenetic imprinting defect of patients with Beckwith-Wiedemann syndrome born after assisted reproductive technology is not restricted to the 11p15 region. J Med Genet 2006;43:902–907.

I. Karen Temple
Wessex Clinical Genetics Academic Group
Princess Anne Hospital
Coxford Road, Southampton SO16 5YA (UK)
Tel. +44 2380 796 170, Fax +44 2380 794 346, E-Mail ikt@soton.ac.uk

Shield JPH, Scharfmann R (eds): Development of the Pancreas and Neonatal Diabetes.
Endocr Dev. Basel, Karger, 2007, vol 12, pp 124–137

The Physiology and Clinical Management of Glucose Metabolism in the Newborn

Kathryn Beardsall · David Dunger

Department of Paediatrics, University of Cambridge, Addenbrooke's Hospital NHS Trust, Cambridge, UK

Abstract

The role of the pancreas and insulin secretion in utero is to support fetal growth and preparation of the fetus with the nutritional reserves to maintain glucose homeostasis after birth. Adaptation at birth includes dramatic endocrine changes, up-regulation of enzymes critical for gluconeogenesis and preparation for the infant to regulate glucose control in the setting of an intermittent enteral supply of nutrition. Disorders of glucose homeostasis are not uncommon at this time, particularly in the setting of prematurity and very low birth weight (VLBW <1,500 g). Although historically hypoglycaemia has been the clinical concern, hyperglycaemia is also a well-documented problem, particularly during the first week in VLBW infants. This hyperglycaemia is a marker of insulin resistance and relative insulin deficiency and may reflect the prolonged catabolism observed in VLBW infants. Reduced insulin levels may also contribute to reduced insulin-like growth factor 1 (IGF-1) generation, and an increased risk of retinopathy of prematurity. Pilot studies of insulin replacement in VLBW infants demonstrate improved glucose control, and increased circulating IGF-1 bioactivity. This suggests that, along with nutritional support, restoration of the normal hormonal balance may be important in promoting anabolism in the VLBW infant.

In healthy pregnancies placental glucose delivery to the fetus is continuous and well regulated in order to meet its requirements for metabolism and growth. The role of the fetal pancreas and insulin secretion is to promote fetal growth as well as ensure there are adequate fat and glycogen stores in late gestation to maintain glucose homeostasis after birth. In utero, the continuous supply of glucose from the mother to the fetus provides the predominant source of energy. After delivery, there is a transitional phase during which the neonate has to rapidly adapt to clamping of the cord, and the delay before an intermittent supply of milk, which is rich in fat and low in carbohydrate, provides an alternative source of energy. During this period, the upregulation of enzymes involved in gluconeogenesis and the association of insulin and incretin secretion with the enteral supply of nutrition are critical in maintaining glucose levels. These changes are under the control of a number of hormones, insulin, cortisol, glucagon and catecholamines. The newborn period is therefore a time when infants are at risk of both hypoglycaemia and hyperglycaemia if the metabolic processes are not activated or regulated appropriately, or appropriate substrates are not available.

Prenatal Glucose Control

Glucose is the primary fuel for the fetus accounting for approximately 80% of energy through facilitated GLUT1-mediated transport across the placenta [1]. The fetal blood glucose level is about 70% of the maternal levels and the GLUT1 receptor is insulin independent [1]. The mother can increase her glucose production by 15–30% in late gestation to provide for the increasing needs of the growing fetus [2]. The expression of the placental glucose transporters changes during pregnancy to facilitate the increased glucose requirements and is also affected by maternal diabetes [3], placental hypoxia, and exogenous glucocorticoid administration [4]. Normally fetal glucose uptake is estimated to range from 4 to 6 mg/kg/min, but in humans saturation of placental glucose transport does not appear to occur until maternal glucose levels are >20 mmol/l.

In a healthy pregnancy, the glucose uptake from the placenta is equivalent to the fetal glucose utilization and fetal liver and kidneys do not produce glucose [5]. Some of the enzymes required for gluconeogenesis are present from the third month of gestation and there is a large flux of lactate and amino acids which could act as substrates for gluconeogenesis [6]. However, gluconeogenesis does not normally contribute significantly to glucose supply and the fetus cannot acutely induce these enzymes in response to hypoglycaemia. In contrast, if there is placental insufficiency or maternal starvation, the fetus is then able to adapt by using these substrates for endogenous glucose production and can also use alternate fuels such as ketone bodies [7].

Glucose not only provides the predominant source of energy to the fetus, but also 40% of the glucose that is taken up is converted to either glycogen in the liver and muscle or to lipid for storage [8]. In humans, glycogen is synthesized from the ninth week of gestation from glucose or lactate, and is stored in the liver, lung, heart and skeletal muscle. Liver glycogen storage increases throughout gestation but mostly occurs in the third trimester, and by term stores are 2–3 times the adult levels [8]. Energy is also stored, predominantly in the third trimester, as fat in adipose tissue with the fat mass in the human fetus at term being 16% [9]. The human placental transport of free fatty acids is not sufficient to account for the amount of adipose tissue that is accumulated and therefore triglycerides must be synthesized from glucose. If glucose supplies are limited, there will therefore be a reduction in both adipose tissue and glycogen stores.

Insulin and glucagon do not cross the placenta, therefore levels detected in the fetal plasma are dependent on secretion from the fetal pancreas. Glucose appears to be the primary regulator of insulin secretion in utero with insulin levels having a positive correlation with plasma glucose [10]. In humans immature endocrine cells appear as early as 10 weeks of gestation, but the main phase of islet differentiation and development occurs in the second trimester. Insulin secretion then increases during the last trimester of pregnancy and is critical for normal growth of the fetus in late gestation [5, 10, 11]. The development of endocrine precursor cells is regulated by a number of transcription factors and proliferation and differentiation of β-cells is dependent on a number of growth factors including insulin-like growth factors as well as cortisol [12, 13]. Increased insulin concentrations lead to increased rates of protein synthesis and increased glucose uptake supporting the role of insulin as a growth-promoting factor [14]. The high insulin/glucagon ratio also appears to be important in maintaining glycogen synthesis and suppressing gluconeogenesis during fetal life.

The important role of glucose and insulin in growth in the fetus is most commonly demonstrated by the altered growth patterns associated with pregnancies complicated by either maternal diabetes mellitus or placental insufficiency. Mothers with impaired glucose tolerance or diabetes mellitus have high blood glucose levels and this leads to increased glucose gradient to the fetus, increased transport of glucose to the fetus, and increased fetal insulin secretion. This promotes fat deposition and produces the typically macrosomic infant [15]. Insulin also has indirect actions on growth through the positive regulation of insulin-like growth factor 1 (IGF-1) levels, by increasing the cellular availability of glucose [16].

In contrast, in pregnancies complicated by placental insufficiency where there is reduced delivery of glucose to the fetus, this leads to low levels of insulin and reduced growth and fat deposition. Insulin deficiency leads to reduced plasma IGF-1 and IGF-2 [17] which play a key role in regulating feto-placental growth with cord blood insulin and IGF-1 levels correlating with size at birth [18]. The fetal insulin/glucose ratio is lower in small-for-gestational-age fetuses compared to those whose growth is appropriate for gestational age [19, 20]. These abnormalities together result in the typical restricted growth and reduced adiposity of the growth-restricted infant who will also have reduced glycogen stores.

The Transitional Phase

At birth there is an abrupt cessation of the supply of glucose and other nutrients and the infant has to withstand a period of fasting before receiving colostrum or milk. During this time, the infant is dependent on mobilization of fat and glycogen stores accumulated in utero. In normal full-term infants, the cord blood insulin/glucagon ratio remains high. Immediately after delivery, there is a significant decrease in plasma insulin and a rise in glucagon associated with increases in catecholamines and cortisol levels at delivery. The stresses of birth, which include transient hypoxia, cold exposure and cord cutting (which increases fetal exposure to catecholamines as they are cleared by the placenta in utero), lead to dramatic increases in catecholamine levels [21]. Infusion of exogenous catecholamines in sheep models decreases plasma insulin and at high levels increases glucagon leading to increased plasma glucose [22]. The elevated glucagon and noradrenaline levels may activate adenylate cyclase which causes an increase in intracellular cyclic AMP and promotes glycogenolysis, lipolysis and gluconeogenesis. Glucocorticoids also promote lipolysis and protein breakdown increasing the availability of gluconeogenic substrates.

Glycogenolysis is critical in maintaining glucose levels immediately after delivery; however, liver stores are exhausted after 12 h and gluconeogenesis is then essential in maintaining glucose homeostasis. The low blood glucose levels and increased cortisol levels at birth stimulate hepatic glucose-6-phosphatase activity. Hepatic glucose-6-phosphatase activity in humans is low before birth [23] and activity rises rapidly after birth in term infants reaching adult values by about 3 days of age [24]. In addition, reversal of the insulin/glucagon ratio through reduction in insulin levels induces PEPCK which is the rate-limiting enzyme in hepatic gluconeogenesis. The concentration of PEPCK continues to increase during the first 2 weeks after delivery regardless of gestational age. Together these adaptations lead to increased hepatic glucose release from gluconeogenesis to maintain glucose supply to vital organs in the newborn infant.

The role of insulin in these postnatal adaptations is unclear as insulin levels decline at birth and there may be a period of transient hypoinsulinism. In fetal life, there is a balance between β-cell replication, neogenesis and apoptosis but at birth there appears to be a transient wave of β-cell apoptosis. Animal studies have suggested that this may occur in rats between 9 and 16 days postnatally or at weaning [25]. Similarly there is some post-mortem evidence of β-cell apoptosis in humans with a new population of β-cells compensating for the perinatal β-cell loss [26]. This may be important in reflecting the change from continuous placental glucose transport to the enteral supply of nutrients. The secretion of incretins may be important in creating a new cell population that is non-proliferative and better suited to metabolic control in postnatal life. Any interference with this process of remodelling may have a critical impact on the ability of the pancreas to meet requirements for insulin secretion in later life. In rats, this period of apoptosis occurs at the same time as a significant fall in the levels of IGF-2 expression [27], and where overexpression of IGF-2 leads to a reduction in the level of apoptosis suggesting a protective role of IGF-2 [28].

Newborn

Although insulin also has a role in early growth, in the perinatal period the primary role of insulin is the maintenance of glucose control. Brain glucose utilization is insulin independent, and glucose homeostasis is important in maintaining glucose supply preferentially to the neonatal brain. Steady-state glucose utilization/production in the term newborn is 2- to 3-fold higher than in the adult (relative to body weight) at 4–6 mg/kg/min [29]. This is in part due to the higher brain/body weight ratio (13% in the newborn vs. 2% in the adult). Glucose utilization may also be increased due to hypoxia, hyperinsulinaemia, respiratory distress or cold stress.

Postnatally insulin secretion is under the influence of neural, neuro-endocrine and entero-endocrine mechanisms: coupling insulin secretion with the enteral supply of milk and release of incretins. Animal studies have revealed the newborn's response to administration of glucose to show a lag insulin secretion with a delayed peak [30], and in the human newborn pro-insulin may be disproportionately elevated [31]. Growth hormone (GH) levels are initially high and the infant shows a paradoxical rise in GH after glucose infusion; the physiological role for GH at this time is unclear. Although the role of insulin is predominantly one of glucose homeostasis, at the same time it remains important in optimizing growth both directly and indirectly through the actions of IGF-1 [32].

In the normal term newborn, blood glucose levels vary greatly compared to the tight glucose control found in adults ranging from 40 to 100 mg/dl [33], and there remains significant controversy over the definitions of both hypoglycaemia and hyperglycaemia. This is in part due to the fact that hypoglycaemia occurs in the healthy term newborn as part of adaptation to extra-uterine life and that in the newborn clinical symptoms of hypoglycaemia may be non-specific. On the basis of neurophysiological and neurodevelopmental outcome studies hypoglycaemia in the newborn is usually defined as blood glucose less than 2.6 mmol/l [34, 35]. In this setting, the neonatal brain can use alternative fuels such as ketones and lactate and is therefore resistant to the low glucose levels [36]. Hepatic ketogenesis markedly increases during the first 24 h after delivery and term infants have a high turnover rate (12–22 μmol/min) with high ketone body concentrations [29, 36]. However, in premature or low-birth-weight infants with limited availability of alternative fuels or altered metabolism such levels may be considered too low.

Although in utero and in healthy term infants blood glucose levels are rarely >7 mmol/l, most neonatologists would not treat blood glucose levels until they were >10–12 mmol/l. Hyperglycaemia is by some considered to be a normal physiological response to stress. However, evidence from preterm studies shows that hyperglycaemia is a significant risk for short-term mortality and morbidity and adult intensive care studies have shown that tighter glucose control may be important in improving clinical outcomes [37].

Very-Low-Birth-Weight Infants

Very-low-birth-weight (VLBW) infants are at particularly increased risk of both hypoglycaemia and hyperglycaemia due to the combined effects of immaturity and prenatal growth restriction.

Hypoglycaemia

Hypoglycaemia is common soon after birth in the VLBW infant due to immaturity of the enzymes required for gluconeogenesis, reduced or absent glycogen and fat stores and impaired counterregulatory hormone responses [38]. Furthermore, there are increased energy demands associated with thermoregulation and breathing efforts caused by respiratory distress, sepsis, hypoxia and polycythaemia.

Until an intravenous supply of glucose or enteral nutrition is provided infants are dependent on glucose production from glycogenolysis and gluconeogenesis. As glycogen stores are predominantly acquired in the third trimester, VLBW infants, especially those who are growth restricted, will have limited glycogen stores. As preterm infants are not exposed to the normal increasing cortisol levels towards term, there may be delayed maturation of the gluconeogenic pathways at birth and the activity of glucose-6-phosphatase has been reported to be low in preterm and small-for-gestational-age infants [39, 40]. Even when these infants demonstrate the metabolic pathways for gluconeogenesis [41], the limited reserves of fat make these infants susceptible to hypoglycaemia [42]. Substrates such as alanine, and lactate are used as alternative substrates and the lower the gestational age and weight of the infant the higher the relative proportion of glucose formed from proteolysis (alanine) [43]. Ketogenesis is also severely limited in VLBW infants due to the lack of fat stores and this lack of alternative fuels make VLBW infants more susceptible to the effects of hypoglycaemia [36].

Hyperglycaemia

Within 2–3 days of life, and usually when on minimal glucose support, hyperglycaemia often develops with the prevalence being reported to be between 20 and 86% depending on the definition [44]. The causes are multifactorial and related to the problems of prematurity and growth restriction, compounded by the physiological response and interventions that occur as part of intensive care. The adverse effects of hyperglycaemia include increased risk of sepsis (bacterial as well as fungal) and osmotic diuresis with subsequent electrolyte imbalance leading to hyperosmolarity which is associated with increased risk of intraventricular haemorrhage [45].

Prematurity itself may be associated with immaturity of the β-cells and thus an inability to produce sufficient insulin leading to hyperglycaemia. In utero studies suggest that there is a consistent increase in insulin levels towards term [19]. However, studies in the newborn have shown that plasma glucose and insulin levels are

Table 1. Pro-insulin, insulin, C-peptide, glucagon levels and insulin/glucagon ratio (median and range) in hyperglycaemic preterm, non-hyperglycaemic preterm and full-term neonates

	Pro-insulin mU/l	Insulin mU/l	C-peptide nmol/l	Glucagon pmol/l	Insulin/ glucagon
Hyperglycaemic preterm	39.9[a, b]	9.4[b]	1.6[b]	146[c]	2.0[b]
(n = 15)	16.9–63.7	2.3–27.3	0.37–3.3	84–481	0.24–7.7
Non-hyperglycaemic preterm	20.75[b]	8.6[b]	1.1[b]	104[c]	2.0[b]
(n = 12)	11.1–33.5	5.2–23.3	0.56–4.3	78–409	0.42–7.2
Full-term neonates	15.9	2.5	0.52	224	0.42
(n = 19)	8.5–66.4	0.6–13.2	0.20–2.7	53–624	0.033–2.6

In both preterm groups, gestational age was less than 30 weeks. Blood samples were obtained in the hyperglycaemic group when capillary glycaemia was found at least twice above 11 mmol/l, before insulin infusion was started. In both other groups, blood samples were collected during the first week of life. Taken from Mitanchez-Mokhtari et al. [31].

[a] Significantly higher than in non-hyperglycaemic preterms ($p = 0.006$).

[b] Significantly higher than in full-term neonates ($p < 10^3$).

[c] Significantly lower than in full-term neonates ($p = 0.028$).

higher in preterm than in term infants [31, 46]. It appears that in hyperglycaemic preterm infants the pancreatic cells are sensitive to changes in blood glucose but respond by increasing secretion of non-processed pro-insulin [31]. Pro-insulin is 10-fold less active than mature insulin and is not able to control blood glucose levels. This pro-insulin may also explain the very variable insulin levels and poor relationship between glucose and insulin levels often reported in the newborn, as some assays may not adequately distinguish insulin from pro-insulin.

VLBW infants are often also small for gestational age and some animal studies have shown growth restriction to be associated with reduced β-cell mass [47]. These changes seem dependent on the model and timing of growth restriction [48] and human data is poor. In utero studies show small-for-gestational-age infants to have a relative insulin deficiency [19]. However, in the newborn insulin levels may be high in keeping with insulin resistance.

There is good evidence for partial insulin resistance in VLBW infants as even when using specific assays insulin levels appear higher than those in term infants (table 1) [31]. Hepatic insulin resistance leads to failure to suppress endogenous glucose production despite hyperglycaemia and raised insulin levels [49]. Additionally, insulin-sensitive tissues such as adipose tissue and skeletal muscle are less abundant in preterm infants than term infants leading to less peripheral glucose uptake [50].

In the preterm infant, there is also a delay in the normal establishment of enteral feeds and the provision of glucose via the intravenous route means that the normal postnatal association of nutritional delivery with stimulation of incretins does not occur. The role for incretins in the newborn has not been well studied but in adults it is clear that incretins play an important role in augmenting insulin secretion post-prandially [51]. In the preterm infant, glucose control improves once enteral feeds have been established and the lack of enteral stimulation may add to the relative insulin deficiency.

The role of GH in the newborn is not clear, as growth at this time is not GH dependent; however, levels are high. There is evidence that in the newborn GH secretion is related to insulin and may be entrained on feeding with an increase in GH in response to hyperglycaemia being a signal for protein synthesis. However, small-for-gestational-age compared to appropriate-for-gestational-age infants have raised baseline GH levels and an increased pulsatility profile, similar to that seen in fasting, and it is thought that this may indicate a role for GH in regulating lipolysis [52].

The interventions required during intensive care and pathophysiological disturbances such as sepsis and necrotizing enterocolitis add to the problems of glucose control in the VLBW infant. Hyperglycaemia may be linked to excess hyperalimentation and drug treatments such as steroids or methylxanthines; however, in the VLBW population it usually occurs independently of any of these interventions. Respiratory failure and sepsis increase the levels of catecholamines, cortisol and GH, which further stimulates glucose release and lipolysis as well as increases insulin resistance. Conditions such as sepsis and necrotizing enterocolitis lead to increased levels of inflammatory markers and pro-inflammatory cytokines like tumour necrosis factor α, interleukin 1 and interleukin 6 cause changes in the insulin receptor signalling, inducing hepatic insulin resistance as well as insulin resistance in both muscle and adipose tissue.

Glucose Monitoring in the VLBW Infant

Although hyperglycaemia is reported to be more prevalent in the VLBW population, data is typically dependent on intermittent blood sampling, 'as clinically indicated', often resulting in many hours between measurements. However, in adults and children with diabetes continuous glucose monitoring is increasingly being used to obtain a clear picture of glucose control throughout a 24-hour period [53]. These methods have recently been validated in the VLBW infant [54]. The continuous glucose monitoring system comprises a disposable glucose oxidase-based platinum electrode sensor that catalyzes interstitial glucose generating an electrical current every 10 s, which is recorded via a cable by a pager-sized monitor. The data cannot be viewed in real time and therefore the monitor is a useful research tool as results cannot impact on clinical care. The sensors were well tolerated by these small infants with no apparent discomfort or problems of infection or oedema at the sensor site. Using this device it was possible to demonstrate that these infants had prolonged periods of hyperglycaemia and periods of undetected hypoglycaemia (fig. 1) [54].

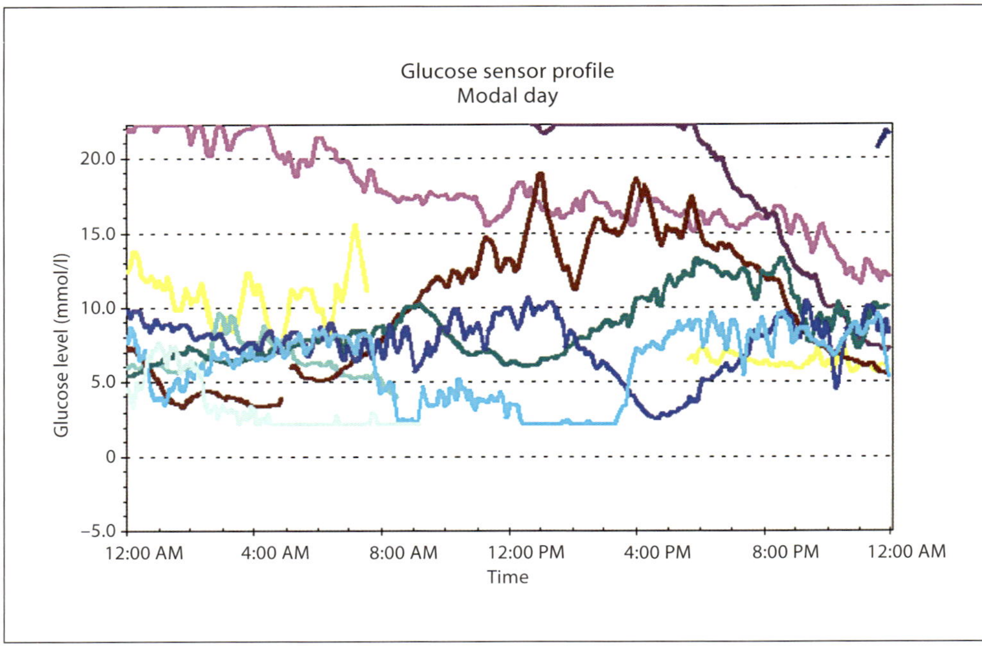

Fig. 1. Profile of glucose control using the continuous glucose monitoring system. Each line represents a separate day on which glucose was monitored.

Clinical Importance of Hyperglycaemia

Recent retrospective studies have shown hyperglycaemia to be a risk factor for short-term mortality [55–57] and morbidities such as retinopathy of prematurity in the premature infant [58, 59]. Hyperglycaemia as a marker of relative insulin deficiency may also have a significant impact on growth and metabolism in the newborn. The reduced insulin secretion with impaired IGF-1 production may create a state of growth retardation and catabolism ex utero. Hyperglycaemia itself has been linked to retinopathy of prematurity in VLBW infants [58] and low IGF-1 levels have been linked to both poor head growth and an increased risk of retinopathy of prematurity [60, 61]. Low levels may also impede pancreatic development, reducing the total β-cell mass.

A large randomized controlled trial published by Van den Berghe et al. [37] in 2001 showed that the prevention of hyperglycaemia in the adult intensive care population by the use of early insulin dramatically reduced both mortality and morbidity. There was a 32% reduction in mortality as well as a halving of the incidence of bacteraemia and a reduction in the number of patients requiring long-term intensive care [37]. Since these studies there has been much debate about the relative importance of the actions of insulin itself compared to the effect of preventing hyperglycaemia [62]. However, no prospective studies had been performed examining the potential bene-

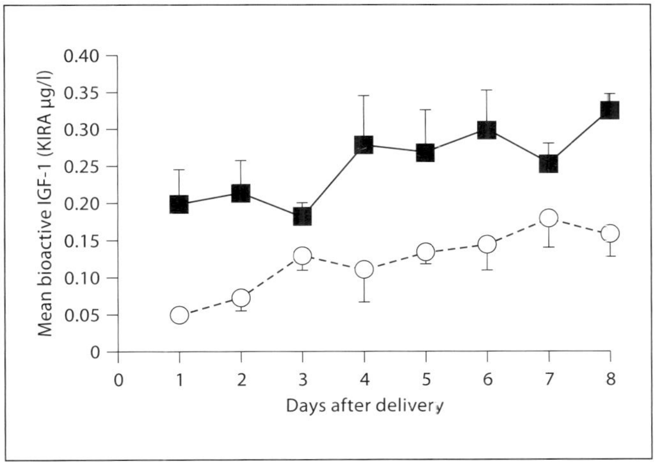

Fig. 2. Median IGF-1 bioactivity (kinase receptor activation, KIRA) during the first week of life in the elective insulin (■) and standard care (○) newborns. Error bars represent 1 SE. Over the whole 7-day study period, average values for IGF-1 bioactivity (p = 0.005) showed significant between-group differences. Taken from Beardsall et al. [69].

fits of early insulin in preventing hyperglycaemia in the VLBW population, and the use of insulin on many neonatal units has been limited due to concerns about the risks of hypoglycaemia [63]. Preterm infants often have an unpredictable response to insulin infusions; however, retrospective studies and a few small prospective studies have suggested that insulin therapy in already hyperglycaemic infants can improve glucose tolerance and weight gain [64–67].

Prospective Interventional Studies in VLBW Infants

In 2007, we reported results of a pilot study to test the hypothesis that early elective insulin therapy with dextrose support would improve blood glucose levels, and promote anabolism in VLBW infants receiving neonatal intensive care [68]. Prevalence of hyperglycaemia and hypoglycaemia were continuously monitored throughout the first 7 days of life using the Minimed continuous glucose monitoring system. The intervention group received a fixed dose of intravenous insulin infusion (0.025 U/kg/h), started within the first 24 h of birth, after confirming that the blood glucose was >3.5 mmol/l (63 mg/dl). The dose of 0.025 U/kg/h was chosen to be half the standard insulin treatment dose for hyperglycaemia in this population, to minimize the risk of hypoglycaemia. Dextrose 20% was also prepared, but only commenced if the blood glucose fell to <4.0 mmol/l (72 mg/dl).

During the 7-day study period there was a reduction in the time spent hyperglycaemic (>10 mmol/l) from 35.9 to 7.6% in the control and intervention groups, respectively (p = 0.035). Importantly the prevalence of hypoglycaemia defined as glucose levels of <2.6 mmol/l (<47 mg/dl) by the continuous glucose monitoring system was no higher in the elective insulin group (0.2%) than in those receiving standard care (0.4%). Interestingly, at the end of the first week, both groups had received similar amounts of insulin and dextrose. However, the early insulin infants also had a 2.4-fold increase in IGF-1 bioactivity compared with standard care infants (p = 0.005) (fig. 2). The increased levels of IGF-1 may explain the improvements in glucose control, despite similar amounts of insulin being infused, as IGF-1 lowers blood glucose levels by increasing peripheral glucose uptake and glycogen synthesis as well as suppressing hepatic glucose production.

We also used knemometry to assess growth during the first week. This method has been validated for use in the preterm infant to demonstrate differences in growth rates over 2 days [68]. We found faster leg length growth in the elective insulin group compared with those receiving standard care [rate of growth 0.74 mm/day (0.37–1.37) vs. –0.38 mm/day (–1.46 to 1.02); p = 0.49]. These provisional results suggest that early elective insulin may have a positive effect on energy balance.

However, in a small pilot study it is not possible to assess effect on clinical outcomes. A larger multicentre randomized controlled trial would be needed to address the question of the potential role of insulin replacement and increased IGF-1 bioactivity levels in growth, retinopathy of prematurity and neurodevelopment. Improving postnatal growth in preterm infants is itself known to be beneficial for long-term neuropsychological outcome but is often difficult to achieve in the VLBW infants despite optimizing nutritional support.

Therefore, these studies have been extended through the NIRTURE Study (Eudract number: 2004-002170-34). This trial is a European-based multicentre randomized controlled trial of early insulin replacement in VLBW infants. The protocol follows that of the pilot study in comparing the infusion of a fixed dose of insulin (with 20% dextrose support), within 24 h of delivery and for the first week of life, to standard care. All infants are monitored with continuous glucose monitoring for the first 7 days of life. The primary outcome will be mortality by the expected date of delivery. Secondary outcomes include rates of sepsis, retinopathy of prematurity and effects on growth. Longer-term outcomes also include insulin sensitivity and neuropsychological outcome at 2 years. The study so far has recruited more than 350 babies. Early results indicate that therapy is efficacious in reducing levels of hyperglycaemia, and may result in greater intake of calories, without excessive fluid administration.

Glucose homeostasis in the newborn is a complex process involving many developmentally regulated metabolic processes. In VLBW infants, immaturity combined with the 'alien nature' of intensive care often lead to difficulties in controlling blood glucose. Further studies are needed to understand better the pathophysiology and consequences of both hypoglycaemia and hyperglycaemia at a time that is equivalent to the third trimester in utero, as this may well have consequences on growth and metabolism beyond the neonatal period.

References

1 Illsley NP: Glucose transporters in the human placenta. Placenta 2000;21:14–22.

2 Boden G: Fuel metabolism in pregnancy and in gestational diabetes mellitus. Obstet Gynecol Clin North Am 1996;23:1–10.

3 Gaither K, Quraishi AN, Illsley NP: Diabetes alters the expression and activity of the human placental GLUT1 glucose transporter. J Clin Endocrinol Metab 1999;84:695–701.

4 Baumann MU, Deborde S, Illsley NP: Placental glucose transfer and fetal growth. Endocrine 2002;19:13–22.

5 Hay WW Jr, Sparks JW: Placental, fetal, and neonatal carbohydrate metabolism. Clin Obstet Gynecol 1985;28:473–485.

6 Jansson T, Ylven K, Wennergren M, Powell TL: Glucose transport and system A activity in syncytiotrophoblast microvillous and basal plasma membranes in intrauterine growth restriction. Placenta 2002;23:392–399.

7 Herrera E, Amusquivar E: Lipid metabolism in the fetus and the newborn. Diabetes Metab Res Rev 2000;16:202–210.

8 van Aerde JE, Wilke MS, Feldman M, Clandinin MT: Accretion of lipid in the fetus and newborn; in Polin RA, Fox WW, Abman SH (eds): Fetal and Neonatal Physiology, ed 3. Philadelphia, Saunders, 2003, vol 1, 3, pp 388–404.

9 Bernstein I: Fetal body composition. Curr Opin Clin Nutr Metab Care 2005;8:613–617.

10 Fowden AL: The role of insulin in prenatal growth. J Dev Physiol 1989;12:173–182.

11 Fowden AL, Hughes P, Comline RS: The effects of insulin on the growth rate of the sheep fetus during late gestation. Q J Exp Physiol 1989;74:703–714.

12 Hill DJ, Petrik J, Arany E: Growth factors and the regulation of fetal growth. Diabetes Care 1998;21(suppl 2):B60–B69.

13 Hill DJ, Duvillie B: Pancreatic development and adult diabetes. Pediatr Res 2000;48:269–274.

14 Susa JB, Schwartz R: Effects of hyperinsulinemia in the primate fetus. Diabetes 1985;34(suppl 2):36–41.

15 Ostlund I, Hanson U, Bjorklund A, Hjertberg R, Eva N, Nordlander E, Swahn ML, Wager J: Maternal and fetal outcomes if gestational impaired glucose tolerance is not treated. Diabetes Care 2003;26:2107–2111.

16 Oliver MH, Harding JE, Breier BH, Gluckman PD: Fetal insulin-like growth factor (IGF)-I and IGF-II are regulated differently by glucose or insulin in the sheep fetus. Reprod Fertil Dev 1996;8:167–172.

17 Gluckman PD, Butler JH, Comline R, Fowden A: The effects of pancreatectomy on the plasma concentrations of insulin-like growth factors 1 and 2 in the sheep fetus. J Dev Physiol 1987;9:79–88.

18 Ong K, Kratzsch J, Kiess W, Costello M, Scott C, Dunger D: Size at birth and cord blood levels of insulin, insulin-like growth factor I (IGF-I), IGF-II, IGF-binding protein-1 (IGFBP-1), IGFBP-3, and the soluble IGF-II/mannose-6-phosphate receptor in term human infants. The ALSPAC Study Team. Avon Longitudinal Study of Pregnancy and Childhood. J Clin Endocrinol Metab 2000;85:4266–4269.

19 Economides DL, Proudler A, Nicolaides KH: Plasma insulin in appropriate and small for gestational age fetuses. Am J Obstet Gynecol 1989;160:1091–1094.

20 Economides DL, Nicolaides KH, Campbell S: Metabolic and endocrine findings in appropriate and small for gestational age fetuses. J Perinat Med 1991;19:97–105.

21 Sperling MA, Ganguli S, Leslie N, Landt K: Fetal-perinatal catecholamine secretion: role in perinatal glucose homeostasis. Am J Physiol 1984;247:E69–E74.

22 Fowden AL: Effects of adrenaline and amino acids on the release of insulin in the sheep fetus. J Endocrinol 1980;87:113–121.

23 Burchell A, Gibb L, Waddell ID, Giles M, Hume R: The ontogeny of human hepatic microsomal glucose-6-phosphatase proteins. Clin Chem 1990;36:1633–1637.

24 Hume R, Burchell A: Abnormal expression of glucose-6-phosphatase in preterm infants. Arch Dis Child 1993;68:202–204.

25 Scaglia L, Cahill CJ, Finegood DT, Bonner-Weir S: Apoptosis participates in the remodeling of the endocrine pancreas in the neonatal rat. Endocrinology 1997;138:1736–1741.

26 Kassem SA, Ariel I, Thornton PS, Scheimberg I, Glaser B: Beta-cell proliferation and apoptosis in the developing normal human pancreas and in hyperinsulinism of infancy. Diabetes 2000;49:1325–1333.

27 Petrik J, Arany E, McDonald TJ, Hill DJ: Apoptosis in the pancreatic islet cells of the neonatal rat is associated with a reduced expression of insulin-like growth factor II that may act as a survival factor. Endocrinology 1998;139:2994–3004.

28 Petrik J, Pell JM, Arany E, McDonald TJ, Dean WL, Reik W, Hill DJ: Overexpression of insulin-like growth factor-II in transgenic mice is associated with pancreatic islet cell hyperplasia. Endocrinology 1999;140:2353–2363.

29 Bougneres PF: Stable isotope tracers and the determination of fuel fluxes in newborn infants. Biol Neonate 1987;52(suppl 1):87–96.

30 Philipps AF, Dubin JW, Raye JR: Maturation of early-phase insulin release in the neonatal lamb. Biol Neonate 1981;39:225–231.
31 Mitanchez-Mokhtari D, Lahlou N, Kieffer F, Magny JF, Roger M, Voyer M: Both relative insulin resistance and defective islet beta-cell processing of proinsulin are responsible for transient hyperglycemia in extremely preterm infants. Pediatrics 2004; 113:537–541.
32 Iniguez G, Ong K, Bazaes R, Avila A, Salazar T, Dunger D, Mericq V: Longitudinal changes in insulin-like growth factor-I, insulin sensitivity, and secretion from birth to age three years in small-for-gestational-age children. J Clin Endocrinol Metab 2006;91:4645–4649.
33 Srinivasan G, Pildes RS, Cattamanchi G, Voora S, Lilien LD: Plasma glucose values in normal neonates: a new look. J Pediatr 1986;109:114–117.
34 Koh TH, Aynsley-Green A, Tarbit M, Eyre JA: Neural dysfunction during hypoglycaemia. Arch Dis Child 1988;63:1353–1358.
35 Lucas A, Morley R, Cole TJ: Adverse neurodevelopmental outcome of moderate neonatal hypoglycaemia. BMJ 1988;297:1304–1308.
36 Hawdon JM, Ward Platt MP, Aynsley-Green A: Patterns of metabolic adaptation for preterm and term infants in the first neonatal week. Arch Dis Child 1992;67:357–365.
37 Van den Berghe G, Wouters P, Weekers F, Verwaest C, Brunyninckx F, Schetz M, Vlasselaers D, Ferdinande P, Lauwers P, Bouillon R: Intensive insulin therapy in critically ill patients. N Engl J Med 2001; 345:1359–1367.
38 Watterberg KL: Adrenocortical function and dysfunction in the fetus and neonate. Semin Neonatol 2004;9:13–21.
39 Haymond MW, Karl IE, Pagliara AS: Increased gluconeogenic substrates in the small-for-gestational-age infant. N Engl J Med 1974;291:322–328.
40 Hawdon JM, Ward Platt MP: Metabolic adaptation in small for gestational age infants. Arch Dis Child 1993;68:262–268.
41 Sunehag A, Ewald U, Gustafsson J: Extremely preterm infants (<28 weeks) are capable of gluconeogenesis from glycerol on their first day of life. Pediatr Res 1996;40:553–557.
42 Diderholm B, Ewald U, Ahlsson F, Gustafsson J: Energy substrate production in infants born small for gestational age. Acta Paediatr 2007;96:29–34.
43 Keshen T, Miller R, Jahoor F, Jaksic T, Reeds PJ: Glucose production and gluconeogenesis are negatively related to body weight in mechanically ventilated, very low birth weight neonates. Pediatr Res 1997;41:132–138.
44 Ng SM, May JE, Emmerson AJ: Continuous insulin infusion in hyperglycaemic extremely-low-birth-weight neonates. Biol Neonate 2005;87:269–272.
45 Finberg L: Dangers to infants caused by changes in osmolal concentration. Pediatrics 1967;40:1031–1034.
46 Hawdon JM, Aynsley-Green A, Alberti KG, Ward Platt MP: The role of pancreatic insulin secretion in neonatal glucoregulation. 1. Healthy term and preterm infants. Arch Dis Child 1993;68:274–279.
47 Garofano A, Czernichow P, Breant B: In utero undernutrition impairs rat beta-cell development. Diabetologia 1997;40:1231–1234.
48 Alvarez C, Martin MA, Goya L, Bertin E, Portha B, Pascual-Leone AM: Contrasted impact of maternal rat food restriction on the fetal endocrine pancreas. Endocrinology 1997;138:2267–2273.
49 Farrag HM, Nawrath LM, Healey JE, Dorcus EJ, Rapoza RE, Oh W, Cowett RM: Persistent glucose production and greater peripheral sensitivity to insulin in the neonate vs the adult. Am J Physiol 1997; 272:E86–E93.
50 Ogata ES: Carbohydrate homeostasis; in Avery GB, Fletcher MA, MacDonald MG (eds): Neonatology: Pathophysiology and Management of the Newborn, ed 5. Philadelphia, Lippincott Williams & Wilkins, 1999, pp 699–714.
51 Baggio LL, Drucker DJ: Biology of incretins: GLP-1 and GIP. Gastroenterology 2007;132:2131–2157.
52 Ogilvy-Stuart AL, Hands SJ, Adcock CJ, Holly JM, Matthews DR, Mohamed-Ali V, Yudkin JS, Wilkinson AR, Dunger DB: Insulin, insulin-like growth factor I (IGF-I), IGF-binding protein-1, growth hormone, and feeding in the newborn. J Clin Endocrinol Metab 1998;83:3550–3557.
53 Amin R, Ross K, Acerini CL, Edge JA, Warner J, Dunger DB: Hypoglycemia prevalence in prepubertal children with type 1 diabetes on standard insulin regimen: use of continuous glucose monitoring system. Diabetes Care 2003;26:662–667.
54 Beardsall K, Ogilvy-Stuart AL, Ahluwalia J, Thompson M, Dunger DB: The continuous glucose monitoring sensor in neonatal intensive care. Arch Dis Child Fetal Neonatal Ed 2005;90:F307–F310.
55 Hall NJ, Peters M, Eaton S, Pierro A: Hyperglycemia is associated with increased morbidity and mortality rates in neonates with necrotizing enterocolitis. J Pediatr Surg 2004;39:898–901.
56 Hays SP, Smith EO, Sunehag AL: Hyperglycemia is a risk factor for early death and morbidity in extremely low birth-weight infants. Pediatrics 2006; 118:1811–1818.
57 Kao LS, Morris BH, Lally KP, Stewart CD, Huseby V, Kennedy KA: Hyperglycemia and morbidity and mortality in extremely low birth weight infants. J Perinatol 2006;26:730–736.
58 Ertl T, Gyarmati J, Gaal V, Szabo I: Relationship between hyperglycemia and retinopathy of prematurity in very low birth weight infants. Biol Neonate 2006;89:56–59.

59 Blanco CL, Baillargeon JG, Morrison RL, Gong AK: Hyperglycemia in extremely low birth weight infants in a predominantly Hispanic population and related morbidities. J Perinatol 2006;26:737–741.
60 Hikino S, Ihara K, Yamamoto J, Takahata Y, Nakayama H, Kinukawa N, Narazaki Y, Hara T: Physical growth and retinopathy in preterm infants: involvement of IGF-I and GH. Pediatr Res 2001;50: 732–736.
61 Hellstrom A, Engstrom E, Hard AL, Albertsson-Wikland K, Carlsson B, Niklasson A, Lofqvist C, Svensson E, Holm S, Ewald U, et al: Postnatal serum insulin-like growth factor I deficiency is associated with retinopathy of prematurity and other complications of premature birth. Pediatrics 2003;112: 1016–1020.
62 Van den Berghe G, Wouters PJ, Bouillon R, Weekers F, Verwaest C, Schetz M, Vlasselaers D, Ferdinande P, Lauwers P: Outcome benefit of intensive insulin therapy in the critically ill: insulin dose versus glycemic control. Crit Care Med 2003;31:359–366.
63 Hey E: Hyperglycaemia and the very preterm baby. Semin Fetal Neonatal Med 2005;10:377–387.
64 Collins JW, Hoppe M, Brown K, Edidin D, Padbury J, Ogata E: A controlled trial of insulin infusion and parentral nutrition in extremely low birth weight infants with glucose intolerance. J Pediatr 1991;118: 921–927.
65 Binder N, Raschko P, Benda G, Reynolds J: Insulin infusion with parenteral nutrition in extremely low birth weight infants with hyperglycaemia. J Pediatr 1989;114:273–280.
66 Ostertag S, Jovanovic L, Lewis B, Auld P: Insulin pump therapy in the very low birth weight infant. Pediatrics 1986;78:625–630.
67 Poindexter BB, Karn CA, Denne SC: Exogenous insulin reduces proteolysis and protein synthesis in extremely low birth weight infants. J Pediatr 1998; 132:948–953.
68 Keller A, Keller E, Hermanussen M, Vogtmann C: Short-term growth of premature infants treated with dexamethasone assessed by mini-knemometry. Ann Hum Biol 2004;31:389–397.
69 Beardsall K, Ogilvy-Stuart AL, Frystyk J, Chen JW, Thompson M, Ahluwalia J, Ong KK, Dunger DB: Early elective insulin therapy can reduce hyperglycemia and increase insulin-like growth factor-1 levels in very low birth weight infants. J Pediatrics DOI: 10.1016/j.jpeds.2007.04.068.

Dr. Kathryn Beardsall
University of Cambridge Department of Paediatrics
Addenbrookes Hospital NHS Foundation Trust
Hills Road, Cambridge CB2 2QQ (UK)
Tel. +44 1223 763404, Fax +44 1223 336996, E-Mail Kb274@cam.ac.uk

Author Index

Subject Index